C000137373

REST IS THE NEW SPORT

Identify Your Fatigue, Improve Your Recovery, Decrease Your Biological Cost

REST IS THE NEW SPORT
© Jef Geys & Uitgeverij Lannoo nv, Tielt, 2015
D/2017/Jef Geys/Uitgever
Translated to English and adapted by Barbara Backer-Gray
Cover Photo © Sven Coubergs. All rights reserved.

This book or any portion thereof may not be reproduced or used in
any manner whatsoever without the express written permission of the
publisher except for the use of brief quotations in articles or reviews.
ISBN 9789082731002

REST IS THE NEW SPORT

Identify Your Fatigue, Improve Your Recovery, Decrease Your Biological Cost

JEF GEYS

TABLE OF CONTENTS

FOREWORD

Dr. Chris Mertens

"A person with normal fatigue feels tired; a person with abnormal fatigue feels sick."

This book by my good friend Jef Geys deals with preventing and addressing unspecified fatigue. As a physician, I can't ignore the daily stream of patients complaining of some form of tiredness. Fatigue is often accompanied with difficulties concentrating, muscle pains, and trouble sleeping. Often, the end result for the patient is long-term disability, along with deconditioning, isolation and depression.

These debilitating illness symptoms seem to taunt advanced medicine, and many physicians have accepted that a well-defined explanation for a chronic fatigue status won't be available any time soon. I agree with Jef that we must focus our attention on maintaining and securing our energy systems rather than hunting for an external enemy. The long wait for a scientific breakthrough, disappointing treatment results, fluctuations in the experience of the illness, and finally the often unhappy ending led us to focus our attention on the balance between a person's energy load and capacity.

Even though every physician knows of cases where energy disruption occurs acutely, most cases are more a matter of an accident waiting to happen. Precisely because, as a primary physician, I have the privilege of following patients over the course of decades, I can now almost effortlessly say who is in for abnormal fatigue. Chronic fatigue doesn't come out of the blue, after all.

We've all been there: right in the middle of an exhausting period, you're dealt yet another blow, so you can't take a break and you certainly can't relax.

But you're determined--you want to take care of these things. You work even harder, sleep even less, and weekends aren't what they used to be, either. So, it begins. You go into overdrive. If this keeps up and you don't take time to recover, chronic fatigue sets in.

Despite your tired appearance, your body tends to show signs of the opposite--a certain restlessness or tension. You might have an elevated heart rate, heart palpitations, trembling, or painful muscle spasms all over your body, and you might have trouble sleeping. These are without exception symptoms of hyper-sensibility to adrenalin, the hormone that gets you moving when you're stressed or when you need to take on a heavy task. However, it doesn't help when you try to carry out the normal day-to-day activities. I believe this is where an explanation can be found for many non-medical fatigue complaints.

So, we need to investigate the delicate balance between energy capacity and load. You'd think it would be easy to determine the daily burden on our energy systems. It's relatively easy to assess whether you had a hard day, exerted yourself intensely, had a few nights of little sleep, or experienced a stress-inducing event. Nobody would be surprised if you had to recover from any of the above. It becomes more complicated, however, when you no longer recover from seemingly normal exertion--when you get up tired, and a weekend or a vacation is no longer sufficient to make up for this fatigue. This is where capacity comes in. This is harder to assess, let alone to measure, and it fluctuates--sometimes you recover successfully, sometimes not so much. But this is also the good news. By pinpointing your individual sensibilities, you can work on increasing your individual capacity.

Jef's powerful approach stems from these very observations. Coming to these insights has been an organic development. It's the result of treating people with prolonged, abnormal fatigue for years, and of many discussions with colleagues about the issue.

Having read this book, I now understand even better what goes wrong in my body. Jef describes in detail how simply making some small adjustments to the way you exercise and train can get your energy store under control, allowing you to acquire optimal, life-long fitness. When I applied it to myself--when I started jogging a little slower and for shorter distances--I felt more energized. It felt counterintuitive, but there you have it.

Therefore, I am bold enough to call this book a real eye-opener. Everyone should read it. It departs from existing scientific achievements, and offers us creative, daring solutions. The system is useful for everyone--from professional athletes who are out of shape to the chronically sick who lack the energy to regain any quality of life. I, for one, have learned that condition and fitness are not the same thing. Anyone can peak after a game or a critical business meeting--it's often the little mistakes that rob us of our energy.

After reading this book, you'll know not to make those mistakes anymore.

INTRODUCTION

As a twenty-year-old, promising competitive cyclist, my motto was, "the harder I train, the better I become". It was all or nothing--I would either get the opportunity to build a professional cycling career or I would continue my studies. It ended up being the latter, because in 1996 I had to discard my motto.

It must have been around the end of March. Until then my best result in young-talent races had been seventh place. This was the first time I made it to the finale. In other classic races like the Tour of Flanders I was usually one of the 20 to 25 cyclists to detach from the larger group toward the end, forming a second group following the leaders. In such races, I usually finished around fifteenth place. But this year would be different. I trained like crazy, behind the motorbike or the car. I trained in the mountains, solo or with cyclists who shared my views on training.

As early as 1993 I bought an activity tracker. In the locker room, other cyclists laughed and joked that, during the race, my watch would probably tell me to slow down because my heartbeat was too fast. I paid them no mind--I gathered data about my races. Back then it was hard to find a trainer experienced in putting together bike training sessions based on the heart rate monitor. So, there I was with my gadget and my data and no idea what to do with it all.

Training was never a chore for me. I was pretty much the champion of training. Even when I was doing well, I still went all out during training, so it wasn't unusual for me to run out of steam before the finish. But I persevered, I did whatever it took. If I didn't do so well in one race, I trained extra hard for the next one. After all, "the harder I train, the better I become", right?

Several beautiful race classics were coming up, The Tour of Flanders, the Flemish Districts Circuit, and a few others. This was going to be it. I felt confident because I had trained like a fiend. I visited my sports physician every two weeks to give him my race results. He did regular blood tests so we could make precise adjustments to my vitamin supplements.

At last, the Sunday of the Tour of Flanders. There had been a kermesse in Meerhout, practically in my backyard, four days earlier. This race was 115 kilometers long (about 72 miles), divided into fifteen rounds of about eight kilometers (five miles) along major roads. The peloton had almost a hundred participants, which made it an easy ride in the group. Up until the halfway mark it was anybody's guess who would win. We cycled along a wide road. I was in the middle of the peloton, which is always easy, yet I felt myself beginning to fall back. This was new! But I stuck with it, even ratcheted it up a notch, completely ignoring my body's signals. Three rounds later I was forced to stop because I had separated from the peloton. My sports physician's verdict? I had over-trained and shouldn't train again for at least two weeks. Goodbye Spring Classics!

This rest period was a new experience for me. Every day I saw my competitors train. I was still convinced that the harder you train, the better you become, so to see them train while I rested was pure agony. But I had no choice. My blood pressure was so low that I regularly felt faint, and deep down I was happy my physician had forbidden me to train even for one minute. Two weeks later, after a general checkup, I was symptom-free. I could sign up for the next race. Without having trained at all, I entered the kermesse in Mol. It wasn't too far from home, and my dad assumed I'd be home soon. He didn't expect me to make it through the first round since I hadn't trained in two weeks. To everyone's surprise, mine most of all, I won the race. From that day on I replaced my motto, "the harder you train, the better you become" with "train hard, rest harder". Or even, "How little should I train to be in top shape?"

I wrote this book to help you in your own quest for a fitter, healthier body. And especially, to adjust your vision on exercise and training. My approach is holistic, acknowledging a clear interaction between mind and body. When you read this book, you will better understand how your body functions in different circumstances. You will also learn to recognize the signs of fatigue, and to adjust your behavior accordingly.

This book is also a guide, with concrete measures for your type of fatigue. Most health regimen books assume you're rested. Based on my own research, however, I must conclude that only thirty percent of the eight thousand test subjects I followed over a twelve-year period are rested enough to participate in such health regimens.

We will start with boosting your ability to recover. Then your body will quickly get back to normal after an exertion, and you will be less likely to develop illnesses. That is the only way to accomplish lasting health.

1.

WHAT IS FATIGUE?

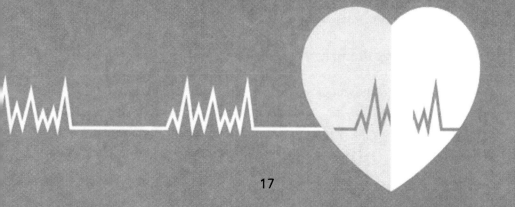

CHAPTER 1:
FATIGUE AND SOCIETY

FATIGUE: EVERYONE EXPERIENCES IT

We all know how it is to feel tired. You feel sleepy and you have no energy or motivation for any activities that aren't absolutely necessary. This usually happens after intense physical or mental exertion or a long period without sleep.

Being tired or stretched too thin is a logical result of your daily activities. Medical literature defines this as a warning sign that you have either reached your limit or passed it. It can manifest itself acutely or chronically. When fatigue occurs acutely, it's usually not a problem. It's normal to feel tired after exertion. Chronic fatigue is different. Feeling tired every day isn't normal or inevitable. And the fact that we all suffer from it doesn't mean you can't do anything about it.

Also, our attitude toward tiredness is historically and culturally determined. Consider the difference in attitudes between the Orient and the Occident. People in the East place more importance on the body's well-being. They understand that you can only be of help to others when you feel rested yourself. Westerners see it differently. We usually give our all to our job, our family and friends, and we only think of our own health after we've taken care of everyone else. That's too bad, because you need to be fit to bring out the best in yourself and others.

WHERE'S THE SUPPORT?

Professional sport and the average person's life both demand a lot of a human body. Yet the two are diametrically opposed. The goal of a professional athlete is primarily a stellar physical performance. This physical aspect is supported by the athlete's mental side. The average duration of a professional athletic career is fifteen years. If you are like most people, however, your mental performance dominates in your daily activities, and your physical side supports it. This is more or less the case throughout your entire life.

Professional athletes' performances are carefully built up. To prepare the body optimally for top performances, they undergo elaborate physical analysis and tests. Apart from their trainers, they have professional guidance from teams of specialists, including sports physicians, osteopathic physicians, kinetic therapists, sports psychologists, masseurs, sport dieticians, chefs, and others.

As a regular person, you're on your own, even though the demands placed on your body can be a lot harder to manage. Even if you're a big-shot executive, on a daily basis you have--at best--a chauffeur and a secretary who manages your schedule. If you're lucky, you can eat at the company restaurant. Wherever you have lunch, though, your options are probably not offered with your optimal nutritional needs in mind.

A professional athlete's daily schedule is planned to the smallest detail (massage, breakfast, training, sleeping, etc.) and it's tailored to his body's biorhythm. Your own life is much less manageable. Appointments run late, kids get sick, traffic jams leave you stressed, and air travel leaves you jet-lagged--there's constantly so much coming at you, both good and bad. Dealing with this emotional rollercoaster requires plenty of anticipation and load capacity. If you have too little of either, you end up running behind and your entire life revolves around your schedule, all of which has consequences for your health.

Yet you visit your primary care physician only once a year for your annual checkup, which is limited to a general health screening, without any focus on physical performance. And it doesn't help that in your (work) environment, the general attitude toward health is: either you're healthy or you're sick. So, you ignore physical warning signs until you are actually sick. Then you go to the doctor, but there's a stigma attached to getting any other kind of support—it's often perceived as a weakness.

If this is the attitude in your particular environment, you have to ignore it. Combining your work and your personal life with athletic performance requires serious attention and guidance. Those who allow themselves (and are able) to be professionally and preventatively supported, understand that their body is an essential element in support of their mental capacity.

It's hard to find institutions that provide comprehensive support for those of us who aren't professional athletes, though. Training and fitness centers primarily support physical performance—they don't have a holistic approach. A professional athlete may well burn up to five thousand calories during a day of training, which clearly justifies fatigue. But if you have a desk job and you burn an average of two thousand calories a day, you're confronted with incredulity when you say that you're also tired at the end of the day. It's important for trainers to understand and create a personal fitness plan based on your specific type of fatigue and its severity.

YOUR SUPPORT STARTS HERE

Since fitness centers focus mostly on one health aspect, we go looking for solutions elsewhere. And to be sure, there's no shortage of programs and philosophies that claim to have the solution. Every day we learn about another silver bullet. Every week someone has found another method or therapy to make you feel better. But these often also come from one focus area (diet, meditation, exercise, etc.), or they don't take the individual into account, let alone your personal fatigue. So these programs are not tuned completely to your needs. This is not to say I don't believe in such methods, but they tend to be too general to result in a targeted, efficient approach. In addition, they often treat the symptoms, not the causes.

Our approach is diametrically opposed to the many health programs promoted everywhere. The solutions offered here were developed after intensively supporting people for fifteen years who suffer from one form of fatigue or another. The approach is holistic, focusing on four areas of the body and mind: diet, sleep, mental relaxation, and exercise. Because looking for solutions in only one of these areas is pointless. Even if an engine is really well-oiled, you can't count on it if you're out of gas.

The goal is to improve your body's ability to adapt after any kind of stressor (travel, work, family etc.) in order to achieve balance--*homeostasis*. Your aim is to reduce your biological cost, and in order to achieve this, you must understand what affects you, how much it affects you and when it affects you. But what is your biological cost? It is the impact of each stressor that knocks the body out of balance, followed by an effort to regain homeostasis. Each stressor on the body activates neural, neuroendocrine and neuroendocrine immune adaptation mechanisms called *allostasis*.

When something's off, it immediately has an effect on your entire system and performance. For instance, simply taking some extra vitamins isn't the solution when you're tired, because your stress doesn't allow your system to absorb more than a fraction of them. And when you don't get enough rest, even a perfect diet won't allow you to perform at your best. You only get the results when you invest in all four focus areas in this approach.

The starting point is *your* fatigued body. So, it's essential to assess both *your* type of fatigue and *your* personal needs because your wishes, priorities and situation differs from those of others. Everyone needs to eat enough vegetables as part of a healthy diet, for instance, but maybe a twenty-minute nap or some recovery training is more important to you.

The solutions offered here aren't quick fixes, but rather an invitation to permanently change your lifestyle. You can only achieve long-term results through long-term effort. Unfortunately, nowadays we are spoiled with immediate gratification in so many areas of our lives. We would all like big results with a minimum effort. No wonder we spend so much on medicines. Real change, however, requires a change in priorities. Of course, you have a lot of responsibilities, but you can only carry them out to everyone's satisfaction if you first take care of yourself.

CHAPTER 2:
STRESS AND RECOVERY

WHAT IS STRESS?

Before we delve into the different types of fatigue, I want to clearly define stress. As you will see, it isn't stress (an external stimulus) that gives you that foggy feeling, but rather your lack of recovery from the normal fatigue that results from experiencing those stressors. And you can definitely change that.

Stress isn't necessarily unhealthy. It keeps you on your toes. It even allows you to up your game every now and again. It stimulates you and gives you the necessary motivation and energy to function at your best. Without stress, there is no competition--the business world, for one, would collapse like a house of cards.

But stress does tire you out and that's where things go wrong. When you don't give yourself time to recover afterwards, stress does become unhealthy and you quickly find yourself in a downward spiral.

The trick is not to *reduce* your stress stimuli, but to *increase* your capacity. You do that by properly recovering from your exertions.

Keep in mind that positive emotions can also evoke stress: the birth of your first child, or anticipating that long-awaited expedition to the Himalayas. Your body can't tell the difference--it responds the same way to positive stress as it does to negative stressors.

YOUR PERSONAL STRESSOR

Stress is any situation your body must suddenly adjust to. A different work schedule, an unexpected traffic jam, or your youngest falling ill--these incidents all require you to adapt rapidly. So, what evokes stress in you is personal, but it is often linked to the unexpected.

A reporter, for instance, is well armed against deadline stress, and a firefighter remains calm in emergencies. But for someone with an entirely different background, these situations would cause anxiety and even panic. For a professional athlete, a one-hour run is a normal exertion while for a beginner the same activity has a much bigger impact on the body. Maybe you're worrying about nothing, but your body still responds the same way as it would if your worries were justified. Stress can be hidden as well, like relationship problems that drag on for years.

Stress is frequently associated with time pressures and responsibilities--twenty pizzas that have to be delivered immediately to a big customer, or you only have half an hour to prepare for a business meeting while you could use a whole day. We're in a constant rat race, chased by the clock. We barely have any time left for fun and when we do, we still experience that same rush-rush feeling. Saturdays end up being just another series of responsibilities and schedules--taking the kids to soccer practice, getting groceries, sending a few quick emails, and then going out with friends. On Sunday, you are up early to train for that marathon, because you're only complete if you're successful in all areas, right? This is how we extend our job pressure to our private life, and before we know it even our down time is exhausting.

We all feel the pressure to "just do it". So, we switch on the automatic pilot. We are being lived. When does it stop? It doesn't, and that's the problem. We don't have time to analyze our lives nowadays. We don't have time to get to the crux of the problem.

And yet stress is not a modern invention. Quite the contrary--it's an age-old defense mechanism. Consider the reptile brain, the oldest in evolution. It's programmed to respond to stress. It responds automatically and quickly upon perceiving danger or aggression.

A reptile in distress has a choice of defense, flight, or disappearing into the background through camouflage. So, a stress response is a healthy, life-saving reaction to everything that can happen to us. It's a physical reaction to stimuli. Fighting or getting away on time guarantees the survival of our species. But evolution didn't take into account that nowadays, fight or flight aren't always options. If you're stuck, if it seems you have no options, or if you ignore your feelings, your stress hormones can't help you. Yet you keep producing them, so your body is on high alert all the time and doesn't switch over to the recovery stage. The stress responses follow one another up and before you know it you suffer from chronic stress. If this situation continues, it makes your life harder and undermines your health.

FATIGUE AND STRESS

We usually talk about stress and fatigue together. Yet fatigue can occur without a stressor. It happens when you burden yourself emotionally or physically without giving yourself time to recover. If you don't get enough sleep, you start the next day on a half-empty tank. And the stimuli coming at you that day still require energy. If you don't do something about this on time, if you go beyond your limits, you end up running on fumes, well on your way to exhaustion. We see tiredness as a weakness--we want to keep our head above water at all times, no matter what it takes. Sometimes it may be wise to take a step back and rest, but we insist on making the extra effort to finish that difficult task. At that moment, your stress hormones take over-- it's the only way you can keep up this demanding situation.

As long as you give your body the time to recover from a hectic period, this approach isn't a problem. But it won't come as a surprise that if you don't step on the brakes every now and then, if you don't refill your tank or even just park your metaphorical car for a while, your tank will soon be empty. Suddenly you come to a standstill--you can't move another inch. You suffer from burnout or you have other chronic fatigue complaints. Counter to what you might think, it's not the stress that causes your fatigue and all the accompanying complaints. It's mostly your lack of recovery.

Although fatigue is not an illness, it does lead to different complaints that can eventually make you sick. If you want to avoid problems in the long term, you must take action against perpetual fatigue.

Long-term problems can include:
- Cardiovascular disease (irregular heart rate, high or low blood pressure, fast resting heartbeat)
- Digestion problems (gassiness, acid reflux, ulcers, diarrhea, abdominal pain, sudden weight changes)
- Psychological problems (apathy, problems concentrating, trouble sleeping, depression)
- Motor control problems (muscle tension, hernias, blockage infections, lower back problems)
- Other problems (burning sensation in your eyes, headaches, ringing in the ears, sinusitis, hoarseness, sore throat, nerve pain, proneness to infections)

SPORTS: THE STRESSOR YOU CONTROL

When we think of stress, we usually think of stress at work caused by hard deadlines, unexpected problems at home or a combination of several challenges. But physical stressors like cardio and weight training also have an impact on your body. A one-hour workout stimulates your adrenal gland, and during extreme exertion you experience other effects of the fight-or-flight response as well, along with sore muscles when you try something new.

It goes without saying, that training for that triathlon, is harder after an already hard day than when you are well-rested. So, running off your stress is not the solution, even if you feel you've been sedentary all day. You may have sat at your desk or counter all day, but the concentration it required still affects your body.

Sure, you feel better for having a two-hour workout in the gym after an exhausting day, but this is only the short-term effect of the adrenalin boost. You may feel that you can handle anything, but that's an illusion. Haste makes waste. It's much better to allow yourself to recover before raising your capacity through training.

THREE STAGES OF STRESS

Canadian-Austrian physician and endocrinologist Hans Selye, renowned for his stress research, defines stress as every physical reaction to a change. Financial insecurity, a family row, illness, an intense physical workout, or pressure to perform all require adaptation. Regardless of the nature of the stress, the effects are the same. His model divides the physiological effects of stress into three stages.

ALARM STAGE

In the alarm stage, also known as the fight-or-flight response, you respond quickly to an unexpected event or threat. Your adrenal glands secrete hormones like adrenalin and cortisol. You literally feel like electricity courses through your body. It happens when you're driving and you suddenly have to slam on the brakes, or when a co-worker attacks you personally and out of the blue. Symptoms of your response in these situations are rapid breathing, increased energy level, and excessive sweating. Since such a situation is intense and your reaction is intense as well, your response immediately affects your body. And it's good to feel this rapid physical reaction, because it means that your body responds quickly in stress situations, which greatly improves your survival chances.

RESISTANCE STAGE
You reach the resistance stage via one of two routes.
The first route is an accumulation of various stressors. Take this worst-case but common scenario: You find out in the morning that one of your children is sick. Finding a solution causes you to run behind on schedule. You leave for work late and on top of that you end up in a traffic jam. You get to work fifteen minutes late, and of course someone makes a remark about your tardiness.

Because of your delay, you're also unprepared for your first task, which leads to another conflict situation. During your lunchbreak, your spouse calls with bad news: you are not getting that mortgage. Later that afternoon your mother calls. Your father has had a fall—he's in the hospital. On the way to the hospital you try to send a text message home, and you have a fender bender. Around 10:00 pm you finally get home, where you get an earful from your better half because they had to deal with sick children on their own.

This example illustrates the accumulation of stressors. It's important to note that these stressors occur both at work and at home--your body can't tell the difference. And even though these are not physical exertions, you nevertheless experience physical stress. To top it all off, many of us then exercise intensely to clear our heads. That's how you inevitably end up in the resistance stage.

The second route to the resistance stage is a weakened recovery ability. In this case your body has a hard time recovering from physical exertion and emotional stimuli. When barely avoiding an accident on the way to work in the morning still affects you in the evening, you know your recovery after a stressor is very low. You then have a higher risk of ending up in the resistance stage. You're on a continual rollercoaster. You feel fatigued, but only on and off. You might feel fine for three days and not so great the next two days. One good night's sleep is not enough to recover, so you underperform. Yet you don't do much about it. You think the source of the problem is external and you hope the situation will change on its own. Or you overestimate yourself and you keep going purely on willpower. However, when you ignore the symptoms or if you don't recognize them, your body eventually decides to pull the plug. Then you arrive in the exhaustion stage.

THE EXHAUSTION STAGE

Because you're late to acknowledge your physical discomfort, or because you fool yourself, your body decides to give up. Exhaustion, unspecified health complaints, drowsiness, and lethargy begin to crop up. Yet you still have that mental drive, thanks to your sense of responsibility and your passion for your job. You get in the car in the morning, but fatigue hits you before you even get to the end of the street. These physical effects may come with mental complaints like short-term memory loss or excessive emotional reactions. Still, the main cause is physical exhaustion, with a side of mental discomfort.

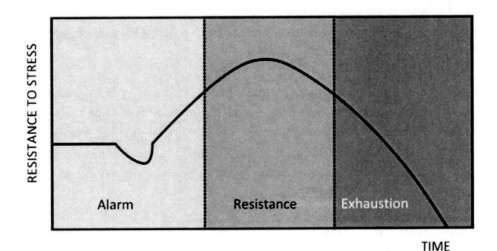

IMAGE 1 The 3 phases of stress

FROM BURN-IN TO BURNOUT

You might be more familiar with the terms 'burn-in' and 'burnout'. They still follow the three stages described above.

In the resistance stage, you're likely to be in the burn-in zone. You drive with your pedal to the metal, you have unspecified complaints, and you build up tension to the breaking point. How long you stay in the resistance stage varies from person to person. The point is, that you always pay for it in the long run in the form of a burnout.

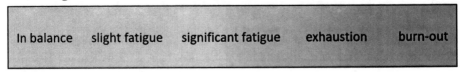

IMAGE 2 From burn-in to burn-out

BEING SICK IS A STRESSOR TOO

Illness is also a sudden, unexpected impulse your body has to respond to. When you have bacterial or viral infections like the flu, your body responds with a fever. This is a good thing-- the rise in temperature is your body's natural defense mechanism against viruses and bacteria. When you have a fever, it's best to stay at home and let the illness take its course. When you tough it out by going to work anyway, or by exercising, you not only infect others, you stimulate your body even more. Exercising with a fever can even cause heart failure, and you could die quite suddenly. Physical exertion with a fever is extremely dangerous--it shows a lack of responsibility to yourself, particularly in combination with stressors such as a draining meeting. Badly healing wounds are also signs that your body's natural ability to recover is at a low level.

Since burnout is the last stage—the stage of complete exhaustion—it's of great importance to detect burn-in on time. You don't get burnout from one night on the town. It develops over months and even years. That's why I encourage you to screen your fatigue and not to give up when your fatigue is abnormal. You might very well have a burn-in that can develop into a burnout. When you get started on solutions while you are still burning in, you decrease the risk of getting a burnout. Unfortunately, a burnout requires a holistic approach, which seldom takes place nowadays-- the physical impact is almost always overlooked.

Image 2 shows the different steps to complete exhaustion:
- Optimal (In balance) = normal recovery ability
- Burn-in (slight fatigue) = your body is going at full tilt--your organs are in overdrive. Complaints range from being vague, mild, and temporary to clear, severe and permanent. If you don't do something your body may decide to crash.
- Burnout = you are burned out, exhausted, and sick

In the following we explore the four types of fatigue you can experience from lack of recovery.

CHAPTER 3:
FOUR TYPES OF FATIGUE

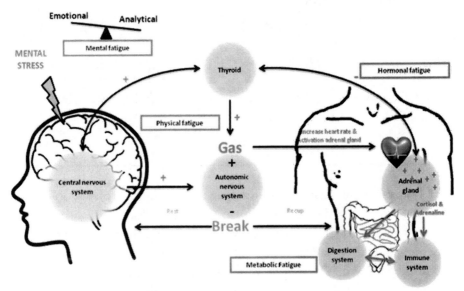

IMAGE 3 The four types of fatigue.

Feeling tired at the end of a day where you have had to process physical exertion, emotional tension, and many different events during the day, is normal. All together this leaves you fatigued in the evening. As long as you recover after a night's sleep, there's nothing to worry about. In that case your fatigue is the sum of the stressors that came at you during the day. How much you can handle depends on your emotional capacity.

Compare this to a checking account, but on a daily basis. Your salary is deposited in the morning. Throughout the day you make payments and you spend money. As a result, you have less money in your account at the end of the day. For some the account is empty and others are even in the red. All this leads to more or less fatigue. Fortunately, you are able to occasionally transfer money from your savings account into your checking account. As long as this doesn't happen too often, there's nothing to worry about. You recover, and the next day you start again with a full checking account. But in the case of abnormal fatigue you have to dig deep into your reserves, and you end up plundering your savings account until you're broke.

That is what severe fatigue feels like. Exactly when you arrive at this stage is different for everyone. We all make different demands of our body, and our situations and expectations also vary. This is why one-size-fits-all health regimens are rarely effective. Your capacity also changes as you get older. Remember your student years, when you got good grades on very little sleep? Despite your lack of sleep, you still felt physically strong and you performed optimally in various areas of your life.

A lack of physical recovery can lead to different types of fatigue.
- In the case of **physical fatigue**, you go into overdrive.
- Prolonged stress leads to **hormonal fatigue**.
- In the case of **mental fatigue**, you have too much traffic in your head, which makes you either block out your emotions or you give them free rein.
- Intestinal discomfort, recurring flues, colds, and metabolic problems often occur after a time of stress. In that case you suffer from **metabolic fatigue**—your energy supply is running extremely low.

Although everyone responds differently, and even though the four types of fatigue can occur together, we will tackle them separately at first. In Part Two we will offer you a recovery plan for the type of fatigue you experience the most. The scientific underpinnings of the four types of fatigue are offered in Part Four.

PHYSICAL FATIGUE

Let's say you have a car that can go 150 mph. To drive at 75 mph, you have to push the accelerator down halfway. But if you don't let your car cool off sufficiently, the next time you accelerate you have to push the pedal further down to make it to 75 mph. In other words, you can still get the same performance, but it requires more energy. When you absolutely must, you can still get up to 125 mph, but you can't sustain it because without enough coolant (recovery) the motor overheats. And you definitely don't get 150 mph anymore. The benefit of a car is that overheating is indicated on your dashboard. To prevent overheating, you slow down.

It's different for our bodies. I notice, for instance, that many people wake up much earlier—sometimes even an hour earlier—than they need to. They set their alarm clock for 7:00 am, but they wake up at 5:30 am. Their body has to wake up earlier so it can be up and running by 7:00 am. Many people stay in bed a while longer though they don't fall back asleep for another hour, at 6:30. The result: they feel dizzy when they get up. Others begin the day at 6:00 am, so at 2:00 pm they have already put in a full eight-hour workday.

In these cases it's normal to experience the classic afternoon dip. Your physical performance decreases, so you reach for caffeine and sugar. These temporarily suppress your fatigue. As long as you stay busy, going from one task to the next while other people are around, you can keep this up. But once you're alone, doing paperwork or reading an article, the physical fatigue sets in and you can barely keep your eyes open. You get home from the day at work, but you're not done yet. You go from one activity to the next. You don't want to get comfortable because you would fall asleep. That makes sense, because your day started at 6:00 am and by 8:00 pm you have been at it for fourteen hours.

This is how physical fatigue insists. As long as you stay busy in an active environment you're fine. But once you're alone, you feel tired, so you take stimulants or engage in stimulating activities to counter the fatigue. However, you're only fooling yourself when you push your fatigue to the background. You wouldn't keep driving an overheated car, would you? It would be much better to take a break in a calm environment. Take a little nap or have a healthy lunch with a good friend. This way your car can cool off.

HORMONAL FATIGUE

Unlike with physical fatigue, in the case of hormonal fatigue your metaphorical car hasn't cooled off completely for a couple of weeks now-- the temperature never falls below 110 degrees. As a result, you start the morning more like a tractor than a Ferrari. Your performance is limited and mediocre. You don't really shift up and there's no way you'd ever reach 150 mph anymore.

How do you experience that feeling during the day? It's important to know that hormonal fatigue is the result of a long drawn out process, in which the balance between effort and recovery has been out of whack for weeks or even months. And yes, you are the cause: you overestimate yourself, you think you can handle more with less recovery, or that you're still twenty. Others blame the situation. It must be the busy job, or your social and family life, which are planned down to the last minute--all situations you feel are beyond your control.

Although trouble sleeping isn't a symptom of hormonal fatigue, your fatigue begins in the morning. You frequently go to sleep too late—around 11:30 or even 1:30—and you no longer need your alarm clock to wake up. Yet you don't jump out of bed upon waking--sometimes you even snooze an extra thirty minutes or more. Anticipating this, you sometimes set the alarm clock half an hour earlier. That way you give yourself that extra thirty minutes. It's a bad idea, because instead of giving yourself an extra thirty minutes of sleep, you actually lose sleep time.

Once you're up, you begin the day in a bad mood. You feel dazed, and it takes you a while to get started. Since you're not really hungry, you don't eat until you're at work. Once there, you head straight for the coffee maker. The caffeine camouflages your sluggishness. Around 10:00 am you're ready to start the day. But still, you need more time than you used to, to finish projects. You prefer to plan standard responsibilities like meetings for the early afternoon. You put off tasks you have to do by yourself, and before you know it you're well into the afternoon, and you've really not done much yet.

Your better work starts in the second half the day, so it's normal that you've only gotten to half of the work by 5:00 pm. Since you feel better as the day progresses, your workdays continue to 8:00 or 9:00 pm. That's when you're on a roll. Twelve-hour workdays are the norm and your coworkers view you as a hard worker. Too bad you only perform half the work because you don't get started until the second half of the day.

In general, you're still able to get excited about opportunities and new challenges, but you no longer care much for the everyday tasks. So, you procrastinate on these--only when you can't avoid them any longer can you muster the necessary energy to tackle them.

MENTAL FATIGUE

Mental fatigue can be compared to driving on a highway. As long as traffic flows smoothly and you can drive at a goodly speed, everything's fine. When it's stop-and-go traffic or a complete traffic jam, however, you suffer from mental fatigue.

Your mental functioning consists of your emotions (reflexes and instincts) on the one hand and on the other your reason (learned behavior). The first five to six years of your life the emotional and reasoning areas of your brain are in perfect balance. From then on three factors determine what happens to that balance and how you respond to situations.

- Your parents: how did they teach you to deal with your emotions? Were you able to talk about them? Were you allowed to cry?
- Your environment: did you grow up in a warm nest? Were you cuddled much? Did you get plenty of attention?
- The circumstances throughout your life, like death and trauma, but also less dramatic events that nevertheless stay with you.

REASON

All actions follow from commands from your brain. The rational part of your brain takes care of planning, organization, decision-making, studying, math, cognition, and absorbing and processing information. It's the cool and collected area of your brain. It's dry, functional, goal-oriented and analytical. It's free of emotions--it's all about knowledge, and the results are preceded by thought processes.

When you're mentally tired, you tend to think it's because your intellect is in overdrive. However, from my personal work experience, I've found that in 75% of cases, mental fatigue is caused by an emotional burden. Think about it: you have the intellectual capacity to properly process appropriate information—you always have. So rationally you do just fine. It's your emotions that trip you up, thwarting your rational ability and causing mental fatigue. And fatigue definitely has a physical impact.

EMOTIONS

Emotion is a feeling you experience without thinking. It's your first and fast interpretation of a situation. For instance, an in itself innocent incident, can lead you to dislike someone or something. Everyone has memories of good and bad teachers. The name of one company makes you smile, while another makes you break out into a sweat, or you get an anxiety attack. Every memory evokes emotions. We experience these situations countless times each day. You're not always aware of them, but they do affect you. This abundance of stimuli causes too much traffic in your head.

Mental fatigue can lead to two different scenarios:
Scenario 1: You're led by reason: you consider all the possibilities and you think everything through, leaving your feelings out of it.

Throughout the years, traumas large and small, stress at school, parental pressure, a strict upbringing, exaggerated perfection, or overstimulation can lead you to lose touch with your feelings. Some circumstances are so painful that they require a sudden evocation of survival strategies, but it's also possible that the pressure builds over the course of years.

When the emotional area of your brain becomes overburdened, a self-defense reflex kicks in and you shut it down. This allows you to live your life on the automatic pilot, because you have to. You must finish your work, you need to take the kids to school every day, you have to pay off your mortgage, you have to have a normal social life.

The result, is that you feel like your life is determined by external factors and that you have little control over it. You're lethargic and you have few intense experiences. You'd rather avoid any confrontation with your emotions because that makes your life more tolerable. If you keep this up for a long time, you lose touch with your emotions. This has enormous consequences for your health, since your body--which is more in tune with your emotions than with your reason--responds to this suppression.

Scenario 2: You're run by your emotions: you're impulsive, you cry easily, you tend to panic, you have irrational fears, etc.

Just as your reasoning can suppress your emotions, your emotions can do the same to your reasoning. In times of intense stress, you no longer respond rationally--your reflexes and instincts take over. That makes sense, because if you'd have to think first about every threat, your survival chances would be seriously compromised. For instance, you instinctively slam on the brakes to avoid a pile-up on the highway. Yet turning off the reason switch can be dangerous, especially in a context without real danger, for instance, when someone personally attacks you out of the blue, or that one coworker refuses to get what you're saying.

When your batteries are properly charged, it's sufficient to just breathe in and out or to lean back to regain control of the situation. But when you're tired, even the slightest stimulus can make you respond emotionally. You have a harder time approaching the situation in a thoughtful and restrained manner. In addition, you're no longer capable of matching your behavior to your long-term goals. Or, in plain English: you do stupid stuff. You overreact or you throw up barricades. You tend to say things you don't mean, and you work yourself more and more into a hole. This can lead to panic attacks, hyperventilation, etc.

BALANCE

Both ignoring your emotions and giving them free range are unhealthy reactions to stressors. An exaggerated control of your emotions leads to insensitivity and being unable to make decisions. People whose emotions reign supreme live life on a rollercoaster. They careen at high speed between extremely varying emotions, from extreme sadness to intense happiness.

It's important to note that people who have a balance between reasoning and emotion don't experience more or less stress. They just handle it better because they're well-rested. They are stable, they have a solid foundation, and they have a lot of self-control. Rather than letting themselves be thrown off by external circumstances and stimuli, they rely on their own inner strength. This is why, they respond less emotionally in tricky situations.

Another thing to note is that mental coaching without insight into your physical functioning can never lead to complete physical recovery. Each emotional stimulus leads to a physical burden. You'll never reach holistic health if you only fix the emotional or rational aspects.

METABOLIC FATIGUE

When you suffer from metabolic fatigue you don't have enough gas in your tank. This can have two causes:

- You lack the energy for the physical and mental activities you enjoy. You don't eat well and you don't give your body the energy it needs, so you're running on fumes, which makes you tired.
- You demand too much from your body. You want to drive a thousand miles non-stop but your tank isn't big enough to hold that much gas. When buying a car, you choose one with a gas tank that fits your expectations for use. To continue the car metaphor in discussing your body: your tank's capacity is not aligned with your expectations as the driver. You either end up in the red or you stop moving altogether.

I do assume you eat enough before you exert yourself physically. Since energy consumption is linked to physical activities, like walking or cycling, you charge your batteries before you exert yourself. This is why, many competitive athletes eat spaghetti before a race.

The sneaky thing is that each stressor has an enormous effect on your energy level, even the stress you experience when you're physically passive. After all, an idling car still uses gas. When you don't rest enough after a sedentary workday, you continue to use energy. If you start exercising in that condition, your energy level sinks even lower. That's when you develop metabolic fatigue. From that moment on you run out of energy sooner, even during basic activities like walking stairs.

CHAPTER 4:
HOW TO RECOGNIZE THE SIGNS

Although fatigue often comes in a combination of the types mentioned in the previous chapter, and even though they influence one another and even exacerbate one another, this checklist will help you determine which type of fatigue you are suffering *primarily*. When you scrutinize your symptoms, try to find the root cause of your fatigue, keeping the main causes and symptoms separate. This way you can pinpoint the areas where you need help. It will lead to faster results. Also, you'll finally know exactly what is going on. Contrary to common belief, physical fatigue can definitely be the cause of mental breakdown.

SIGNS OF PHYSICAL FATIGUE

You're in chronic fight-or-flight mode, though you aren't fully aware of it, thanks to the adrenalin your adrenal glands produce. It's not until you sit back to unwind--when you sink into your easy chair and turn on the TV-- that you feel tired. If you keep this up for a prolonged period, it can also lead to hormonal fatigue. These are the symptoms:

SYMPTOMS WHEN YOU'RE PHYSICALLY FATIGUED
You experience all the aspects of a stress response. Your heart rate, blood pressure, muscle tension and blood glucose all rise, you sweat easily, and your breathing is shallow and fast. Your digestion slows down, your mouth is dry, and you're on high alert. Your pupils are dilated and sometimes your eyes burn. Because your arteries widen, you may have pounding headaches. Sometimes you suffer from neck pain, shortness of breath, chest pain, dizziness, and/or heart palpitations.

In the first stage of physical fatigue you lose weight. In the long run, however, when you're headed toward hormonal fatigue, you actually gain weight. If you have allergies, they can be exacerbated because pushing down on that pedal raises your histamine levels. Histamine is the chemical your body creates during an allergic reaction. As a result, you get skin irritations like itchiness, rashes, swelling, and/or redness.

You sometimes feel tired despite the adrenalin, but you believe this is caused by external circumstances. A sleepless night, stress at work or at home--you think these are the causes of your fatigue.

TRAINING WHEN YOU'RE PHISICALLY FATIGUED

You have a false sense of fitness. The adrenalin allows you to be optimistic at the starting line, but when you have to speed up, you quickly reach your limit. You respond sluggishly, your balance is off, and you perform under your norm. This may be accompanied by torn and sprained muscles.

Sometimes you suffer from muscle cramps or involuntary spasms in your eyelids or calves.

NUTRITION WHEN YOU'RE PHISICALLY FATIGUED

You aren't that hungry—you're fueled by adrenalin. Since you eat so little during the day, your energy level drops once your adrenalin levels drop in the evening. Your high blood glucose levels lead you to crave sugars. Sweets are your way of refilling your tank during a sugar dip.

You keep that gas pedal pushed in, so your body thinks you're in a state of emergency. Very little blood goes toward your digestion, because it isn't a priority in emergencies. And a slower digestion can lead to constipation.

SLEEP WHEN YOU'RE PHYSICALLY FATIGUED

The adrenalin makes you wake up around 4:00 or 5:00 am. You hit the ground running and you sustain that grueling tempo as long as your work keeps you busy. You go from one task to the next. Once the responsibilities are over--during a down time in your day or in the evening after your workday is done--your adrenalin level drops. Your tiredness hits you like a ton of bricks, but even so, you have a hard time falling asleep. On vacation, you are overcome by an extreme sense of fatigue.

MENTAL HEALTH WHEN YOU'RE PHISICALLY FATIGUED

Exhaustion leads to a decreased release of adrenalin, which in turn can hinder the production of the enjoyment hormone dopamine. This can lead to mood swings or crying fits. You reach for stimulants like alcohol, nicotine, sex, or extreme sports.

You're oversensitive to stimuli. Even the faintest light, noise or an inappropriate remark affect you, which is why you sometimes lose control of your emotions.

You can tolerate less from the people around you (your immediate family), and you're oversensitive to what they think, say and do. You get easily upset and sometimes you can be violent, either verbally or physically.

SIGNS OF HORMONAL FATIGUE

Your fatigue is chronic. Your endocrine system—responsible for your hormone production--is messed up and you get your adrenalin via cortisol. Acute stress has given way to chronic stress. Your chronic fatigue and the diminished functioning of your adrenal glands affect your cortisol level. You need cortisol in the morning to wash away the sleep hormone melatonin, but your cortisol value isn't high enough. That makes you feel drowsy. Since you suffer less from acute problems than physically fatigued people, you hope this is a passing phase. In reality you're unable to completely turn off your stress mode--you keep it on standby. You must act fast if you don't want to come to a complete standstill.

SYMPTOMS WHEN YOU'RE HORMONALLY FATIGUED

Your immune system functions at low levels. You need more time than average to recover from illness. This goes both for a flu and a mental low after the loss of a loved one. Wounds and injuries also take more time to heal--infections tend to linger. You might suffer from recurring airway infections such as sinusitis, bronchitis, or a sore throat.

Your blood pressure is low. You experience blackouts and dizziness when you get up from a sitting or prone position. Because of your low blood pressure, you feel weak all day long and you have no energy.

You have a multitude of complaints that come and go without feeling truly sick. One day your digestion might be off and the next day your muscles might be stiff. You feel flabby and bloated.

TRAINING WHEN YOU'RE HORMONALLY FATIGUED

You generally start the workday early and you don't get home until 7:00 pm. Because of this grueling schedule you aren't as fit as you'd like to be. You barely reach your top speed--you chose to run slower but longer. So you exhaust your body twice: first you work too long and then you work out too long.

You suffer from chronic infections such as tennis elbow or a sensitive Achilles tendon. You have a reduced libido.

NUTRITION WHEN YOU'RE HORMONALLY FATIGUED

Since you're not hungry in the morning, you tend to skip breakfast, so you have even less energy. You need caffeine to counteract your morning daze, and you give yourself additional energy boosts with snacks, sweets, and sodas. This leads to weight gain, insulin resistance, and--in the long run—type 2 diabetes.

Your low blood pressure makes you crave salt.

Prolonged stress can damage the mucous membrane of your stomach lining, which can lead to ulcers. Also, bad bacteria can enter your bloodstream, resulting in infections, allergic reactions, and headaches.

SLEEP WHEN YOU'RE HORMONALLY FATIGUED

You sleep through the night, but despite your regular sleep pattern, you never feel completely rested when you wake up. You're also a habitual snoozer. Because of your low cortisol value, you are a slow starter--you feel lethargic during the first hours of the day. You don't start feeling energetic until around 10:00 am and you usually experience an afternoon slump around 3:00 or 4:00 pm. You feel better in the evening. After being awake for twenty-two hours and then having dinner, you get your second wind, and you end up going to bed late.

MENTAL HEALTH WHEN YOU'RE HORMONALLY FATIGUED

You feel apathetic and you tend to procrastinate. You're hard to motivate for general chores and basic activities. They also seem to take ten times as much energy as they used to because it's hard to concentrate.

Because of your deficiency in the feel-good hormones serotonin and dopamine, you experience less joy and happiness. Even things you used to enjoy become a chore. Your work and relationships feel meaningless because of your apathy in the weekend or during other free time. You sometimes wonder if there's still any point. However, new experiences with a wow factor can still get you going.

You're touchy, you fret, and your mood might be affected.

If you're female, you might suffer more menstrual complaints than usual. You feel more fatigued, bloated, and grumpy.

You're absent-minded and your memory isn't what it used to be. Your thoughts are foggy. You have difficulty making decisions, even about simple things, like what to make for dinner or what to wear.

SIGNS OF MENTAL FATIGUE

Both repressing your emotions and letting them rule you stimulates your adrenal gland, which produces stress hormones. You're short-fused with the people around you. A disrupted endocrine system results in a delayed physical recovery, so you increase the risk of fatigue and illness. Even though your emotions are at the core, you sometimes experience the symptoms of physical fatigue.

SYMPTOMS WHEN YOU'RE MENTALLY FATIGUED

You're forgetful and you feel blue. You gradually become more apathetic.

You're oversensitive to stimuli. The least amount of light, noise or an inappropriate remark can throw you off. This extra stress leads to more adrenalin, which is why you sometimes suffer physical fatigue and the accompanying complaints.

TRAINING WHEN YOU'RE MENTALLY FATIGUED

You don't feel like working out any more--you just can't muster the energy. You're the workout procrastination champion. A thirty-minute workout is already too long, though group workouts or activities with a workout buddy can still motivate you. Your reflexes slow down. Car races, boxing, or martial arts are definitely not your thing.

NUTRITION WHEN YOU'RE MENTALLY FATIGUED

You feel blue so you reach for stimulants like alcohol, chocolate, and other sweets.

SLEEP WHEN YOU'RE MENTALLY FATIGUED

You have a hard time getting out of bed because you don't feel like starting the day. You worry non-stop, which makes it hard to fall asleep at night. Your persistent thoughts can lead to disrupted sleep, usually in the second half of the night.

MENTAL HEALTH WHEN YOU'RE MENTALLY FATIGUED

You have trouble concentrating--it often takes you twice as long to finish a task as it used to. You're easily distracted by street sounds, a ringing phone, etc. Your ability to plan and manage your time is severely diminished. You procrastinate. You're touchier toward the people you care about, like your immediate family, and sometimes you lose control of your emotions, at which point you might cry or yell. Toward people outside your inner circle you still manage to restrain yourself and stay polite.

SIGNS OF METABOLIC FATIGUE

Your energy systems don't work like they should because your body has slipped out of balance. You feel reasonably fit in the morning. Your stress hormones prevent you from feeling hungry, so you don't eat much early in the day. As a result, you can feel weak and faint in the evening, especially after physical exertion.

SYMPTOMS WHEN YOU'RE METABOLICALLY FATIGUED

Because you ignore basic needs such as hunger, thirst, and sleep, your body starts to use up its reserves. You experience a general lethargy during every physical exertion and you reach your limits quickly. When you walk upstairs your legs feel weak, and walking thirty feet is already too much. You lack all strength. Even in stress-free situations you sometimes feel off, weak. You're in an advanced state of exhaustion and you need a lot of time to recover your inner balance in order to get more energy.

TRAINING WHEN YOU'RE METABOLICALLY FATIGUED

Your lack of energy leads you to quickly reach your limits during workouts. You develop muscle stiffness sooner than you used to. Not only your endurance, but also your coordination may be off. Your reflexes are slower, leading to more injuries such as ankle sprains.

NUTRITION WHEN YOU'RE METABOLICALLY FATIGUED

You constantly push down on the pedal—it takes all your energy just to get through the day—so very little blood goes to your digestion. Your digestive system slows down, which affects your stomach acid. This leads to an inadequate uptake of nutrients. Your inability to absorb nutrients can lead to deficiencies in iron, vitamin B12, and folic acid. You're now at risk for anemia. Under these circumstances, eating healthfully isn't sufficient to give your body enough micronutrients. You have a lot of waste and toxins in your body.

SLEEP WHEN YOU'RE METABOLICALLY FATIGUED

You have no problem rising in the morning--it's more the physical exertions that are hard because you lack the energy. During the day, you don't have much of an appetite because you run on adrenalin, but you wake up hungry in the middle of the night. When your body doesn't produce serotonin, the precursor of melatonin, you can have trouble falling asleep.

MENTAL HEALTH WHEN YOU'RE METABOLICALLY FATIGUED

You may experience less focus and concentration. Since you don't know what's causing your loss of energy, you start worrying about your health. You want to give your all, but your lack of energy doesn't allow it.

LET'S RECAP

1. **Feeling tired** at the end of the day is normal. All the stressors of the day leave you fatigued in the evening. As long as you recover after a night's sleep, there's nothing to worry about.

2. In the case of **abnormal fatigue**, you don't recover every night. If you don't do something about this on time, if you go beyond your limits, you end up running on fumes, and you're well on your way to exhaustion. Exactly when you arrive at this stage is different for everyone.

3. **Stressors don't cause fatigue**, but rather your **lack of recovery** from the normal fatigue that results from experiencing those stressors. The trick is not to *reduce* your stressors, but to *increase* your recovery capacity.

4. **Physical fatigue** develops when your body doesn't recover from one or more daily stressors, but you keep going anyway, until you exhaust yourself.

5. **Hormonal fatigue** sets in when you have been running on fumes for an extended period of time. You feel sluggish and listless all day.

6. **Mental fatigue** can be caused **by repressing your emotions**. This has enormous consequences for your health, because your body responds to this suppression. If you keep this up for a long time, you can actually lose touch with your emotions.

7. Mental fatigue can also occur when your emotions **suppress your reasoning**. In times of intense stress, even the slightest stimulus can make you respond emotionally. This can lead to panic attacks, hyperventilation, etc.

8. When you suffer from **metabolic fatigue**, you've been running on fumes for a while, and it's affecting your body's ability to absorb

the energy it needs. Your energy levels sink ever lower and you even deplete your emergency supplies.

9. The four types of fatigue influence and exacerbate one another, but in order to work on recovery, you first need to find out **which type of fatigue** you suffer from *primarily*. This way you can pinpoint the areas where you need help.

HEALING HABITS

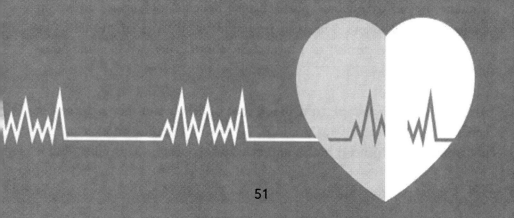

CHAPTER 5: NUTRITION

Many people feel tired after eating. That's strange. It means that what you're eating is a burden rather than a source of energy. Nutrition should increase your energy stores and provide you with the necessary elements for a healthy, balanced and functioning body. In the following we will first discuss the main ingredients of a balanced diet, and then we'll show you how a proper diet can enhance your performance.

MACRONUTRIENTS YOUR DIET'S MAIN COMPONENTS

Proteins, carbohydrates, and fats are macronutrients that can be found in food. They all provide energy.

PROTEINS AS BUILDING BLOCKS

Proteins are the body's builders. They play a major role in almost all physical processes. Proteins consist of various amino acids--organic compounds that are the basis for growth, maintenance, and recovery of your cells, blood, muscles, bones, organs, and nervous system.

Of the twenty-relevant amino acids you need for the creation of proteins, nine are essential amino acids, which means they're not made by your body and must therefore be consumed via food or supplements. They are: histidine, lysine, tryptophan, phenylalanine, leucine, isoleucine, threonine, methionine, and valine. They can be found in all types of proteins. We recommend eating protein-rich food daily, about every two to three hours in meals and snacks.

Amino acids do not impact the blood glucose levels and they reduce your appetite. But do watch your portions, because not getting enough protein undermines your general health and can lead to decreased wound healing and anemia. On the other hand, consuming too many proteins is useless to your body--you just urinate out the excess.

Food	Portion	Protein
Almonds	50 g	10 g
Avocado	1	4 g
Broccoli	250 g	5 g
Kidney beans	100 g (cooked)	7 g
Lentils	100 g (cooked)	10 g
Oatmeal	50 g	6 g
Pistachio nuts	50 g	7 g
Quinoa	150 g (cooked)	10 g
Spinach	200 g (cooked)	5 g
Sweet potato	200 g	5 g
Walnuts	50 g	7 g

TABLE 1 Protein in food

Adults need 1 g protein/kg body weight a day. If you work out a lot, you might consume up to 2 g/kg body weight. Weightlifters even consume 6 – 7 g/kg body weight. This does, however, place a bigger burden on the kidneys.

There are two types of protein:
- Animal proteins can be found in meat, fish, poultry, eggs, milk, and cheese.
- Plant-derived proteins can be found in vegetables (beans, sweet potatoes, and corn), legumes, sprouts, nuts, seeds, mushrooms, and grains. You can also find them in meat substitutes like tofu, Quorn, seitan, and tempeh.

The benefit of plant-derived proteins is that they not only contain a goodly dose of amino acids, but also fiber, minerals, and vitamins.

CARBOHYDRATES AS FUEL

Carbohydrates are sugars. They give you an energy rush. They're found in bread, potatoes, flour, baked goods, rice, muesli, corn, legumes, honey, all sweet beverages, and processed foods. Your body converts these carbohydrates into glucose. Glucose is the fuel for your central nervous system and your physical activities, so you need it mainly during the day.

Carbohydrates give your body a quick energy boost. If you eat too many carbohydrates, your blood glucose levels shoot up, in which case insulin sees to it that the excess is taken from your blood and stored in your liver and muscles as glycogen. Since the storage capacity of your liver and muscles has its limits, any further excess is stored as belly fat.

For optimal energy management, it's best to eat foods with a low glycemic index. The glycemic index is the number that indicates the impact of the food on your blood glucose levels. The lower the glycemic index of a food is, the more stable your blood glucose remains. That's a good thing—it's how you provide your body with a continuous energy stream.

Hence the difference between simple and complex carbohydrates. Complex carbohydrates like whole-grain bread and whole-grain pasta, oatmeal, or brown rice have a low glycemic index. Their fiber minimizes blood glucose spikes and makes you feel satisfied. Simple carbohydrates have a high glycemic index. They cause spikes and drops in your blood glucose levels. As a result, you develop an increased craving for sweets. This can lead to addiction. The insulin spikes—your body's reaction to blood glucose spikes--also cause stress responses in your body.

Nutrients and the glycemic index:

- Low glycemic index: red berries, vegetables, legumes like beans and peas, whole-wheat grains and whole-wheat pastas;
- Average glycemic index: breakfast cereals, pastas, steamed or cooked potatoes, bananas, dried fruit, maple syrup;
- High glycemic index: fruit, rock sugar, honey, candy, jam, syrup, white bread, white rice, fries, baked potatoes, mashed potatoes, chips, chocolate, and alcohol.

Preparation and combinations also impact the glycemic index:
- **Heating** releases the sugars in carbohydrate and transforms them into starch. Therefore, pasta al dente and potatoes baked in the skin score lower than regularly cooked pasta and mashed potatoes.
- Because almonds have **no carbohydrate**, they lower the glycemic index of any food they're added to, like fruit or cereal.
- **Fiber, protein and fat also lower** the glycemic index of foods. Of course, fats do have more calories.
- **Ripe fruit** has a higher glycemic index than unripe fruit.
- **Fermented foods like yoghurt** lower the glycemic index because the natural acid reduces the rate of glucose absorption in the blood.

At least as important as the glycemic index is the glycemic load. This number indicates not only how much a nutrient increases your blood glucose levels, but also the amount of energy per portion. The glycemic index is calculated per 50 g carbohydrate; however, sometimes these amounts aren't feasible. For instance, in order to get 50 g carbohydrate from carrots, you would have to eat more than a pound of carrots. The glycemic load, on the other hand, is calculated per average portion of an ingredient. The lower the glycemic load, the better.

Proteins and fats are digested in your stomach. Carbohydrate digestion, on the other hand, starts in your mouth. That's why it's so important to chew properly. It's also best not to drink anything with your meal, because the additional liquid changes the composition of your saliva, so the digestive enzymes can't mix as well with the carbohydrate.

FATS AS DIESEL
Contrary to what you might think, fats aren't all that bad for you. They supply more protein than carbohydrates and they have no effect on your blood sugar levels. This means that fats are not addictive. However, fat is a relatively slow energy supplier, because it first should combine with oxygen. That means that, in order to lose weight with exercise, you should exercise for medium to long periods and at talking speed (70% of maximum heart rate).

Fats include essential vitamins and fatty acids. They have an important effect on the immune function and they take care of your energy storage, so you don't need to dip into your muscle glycogen for energy. Is this a free pass for daily portions of fries or chips? Absolutely not, because the trick is to eat the right fats.

The three types of fat:
Unsaturated fats are divided into simple (omega-9) and complex unsaturated fatty acids (omega-3 and 6).

Omega-9 fatty acids can be found in olive oil, avocadoes, linseed oil, sesame seeds, peanuts, hazelnuts, almonds, pistachios, cashews, and pecans. They lower blood pressure, they contribute to good cholesterol, and they minimize inflammation.

Do eat them in moderation, because they're high in calories. Since your body produces Omega-9 itself, it's not essential. Opt for a higher consumption of omega-3 instead, a healthy fatty acid with high levels of vitamins A, D, and E.

Especially fatty fish like salmon, herring, and eel are loaded with omega-3, as are omega-3 eggs, hempseed, walnuts, chia seeds, and linseed. Omega-3 and omega-6 can only be found in food. Western food with lots of oil and fat--in other words, most foods you find in the grocery store--usually contains omega-6. it's best to avoid large portions, because they can lead to inflammation. An excess of omega-6 also undermines your omega-3 because they compete for storage in your body.

Tip: Unsaturated fats oxidize quickly when heated, which results in free radicals. That's why it's best to use oils like olive oil and linseed oil cold—and preferably cold-pressed--in salads, or add fish oil in the form of fresh fatty fish: salmon, mackerel or eel. Margarine is also a plant-derived oil—it's best to avoid heating it.

Saturated fats increase your bad cholesterol. An excess is related to cardiovascular disease, diabetes, and cancer. They can be found in animal-derived food products like cheese, butter, fatty meat, and processed meats like sausages. Opt instead for proteins high in unsaturated fat, like salmon, tuna, mackerel, eel, lobster, fresh crab, shrimp, game, steak, turkey, chicken, eggs (one egg yolk and four egg whites), mozzarella cheese, Greek yogurt, soybeans, soy flakes, tofu, or nuts.

In general, saturated fats are solid at room temperature and of animal origins. But some plant-derived fats--like coconut oil, palm oil, and cacao butter--are also saturated fats. Since, other than most plant-derived oils, coconut oil and cacao butter can stand high temperatures, they're your best choice for cooking. They're also better than other saturated fats at breaking down in your liver. If do you opt for butter, go for unpasteurized butter-- the vitamins and enzymes are lost in the pasteurization process. Palm oil is on the black list because it contains palmitic acid, which is bad for your cardiovascular system.

Trans fats are found in margarine, pizza, chips, cookies, sodas like coke, and other ready-made foods. At extreme temperatures these oils, high in unsaturated fats, can lead to the formation of trans fat acids. So avoid processed foods, because they increase your bad cholesterol, and therefore your risk for cardiovascular disease. In addition, these fats weaken your immune function and mess with your metabolism. When you look at the list of ingredients of a food, keep in mind that 'plant-derived fats' 'partially solidified fat' and 'hydrogenated fat' usually indicate the presence of trans fats.

NUTRITION COMBINATIONS: DO'S AND DON'TS

Some nutrients require more energy to digest than others. They also have a different influence on your acid-base balance. This is why, certain combinations can lead to bloating, acid reflux, drowsiness, or a heavy feeling after eating. A fatigued body struggles with a less than optimal digestion and a disrupted acid base balance, so it's imperative to create good food combinations--those that lead to an optimal absorption of nutrients and stable blood glucose levels.

The main thing is to *avoid combining proteins and starchy products*. Starches are mostly slow carbohydrates. Proteins and starches are digested differently, and eating them together can lead to fermentation in your stomach. Bread rolls, pasta, or rice are best eaten without meat, fish or cheese. Legumes contain both proteins and starch, so they are also best eaten separately. Some vegetables also contain carbohydrate, like cauliflower, artichoke, pumpkin, corn, and beets.

Combine protein with leafy greens, fats or fruit. This means that, for instance, meat or fish can be combined with vegetables, or yogurt can be combined with fruit. Almonds are great at maintaining constant blood glucose levels and ideal in combination with fruit.

Foods that contain starch go with leafy vegetables, fats, sugar or fruit. Examples: pasta with vegetables, mashed potatoes, or salads with bread. Oatmeal is best cooked in water--you can add mashed banana, coconut oil and possibly some cinnamon. If you really want to eat granola or oatmeal with milk, opt for almond or rice milk. Other grains and fruit are also good combinations, perhaps with some honey.

Note that these rules help your digestion when your body needs to be in performance mode. If you combine them when you're relaxing, they might bother you less.

DAILY NUTRITION PLAN FOR EVERYONE

Your mornings are busy, so you skip breakfast or you wolf down something in the car. You have an elaborate lunch and an even richer dinner. A good breakfast, however, gives you the necessary energy for the beginning of the day. It's best to end your day with light foods so as not to disturb your sleep. If you want to feel more energetic during the day, have breakfast like a king, lunch like a prince, and dine like a beggar. It's best to eat six times a day--three main meals and three snacks.

General

Simple sugars and sugar you can see (as on a teaspoon for tea or coffee), should be erased from the menu. If you really can't do without sugar, don't use sugar after your most important activity of the day, like a meeting or your workout. Also avoid sugar before you go to bed.

Consider the preparation. Preparation methods can be ranked from good to bad: steaming, boiling, stir-frying, grilling, roasting, baking, and frying. Steaming vegetables is especially good because you lose a minimum in micronutrients in the cooking process.

When you choose fruit and vegetables, go for color--the brighter the color, the better. In the category of red, orange and purple, opt for red beets, carrots, bell peppers, eggplant, pumpkin, tomatoes, blueberries, blackberries, or cherries. Spinach, endive, broccoli, green bell peppers, cucumber, and zucchini are healthy green and yellow vegetables. Vegetables high in sulfur and sharp vegetables are also very healthy: onions, green onions, garlic, Brussel sprouts, broccoli, radish, and peppers.

Avoid overusing kitchen salt, additives, artificial colors, preservatives, or taste enhancers. Opt for natural flavors like sea salt, garlic, onions, lemon, mustard, basil, ginger, cinnamon, turmeric, pepper, real vanilla, and saffron.

Upon rising
Drink a big glass of lukewarm water first thing in the morning to compensate for your nightly fluid loss. Add the juice of half a lemon. That gets your digestive system started, it supports your liver, and it clears up your skin. A glass of water with a teaspoon of honey and two teaspoons of apple vinegar has also been proven to ease digestion, protect colon health and decrease acid reflux. Grapefruit juice may be your perfect ally if you want to lose a few pounds--just consult your health provider because it's contraindicated with some medications.

Breakfast
Breakfast gives your body the necessary energy to start the day. It's also essential for a well-functioning brain, because your brain is an energy hog. A good breakfast helps promote your memory and concentration, because it provides your brain with glucose and fats.

Grains	Topping	Flavoring
Spelt boiled in water	yoghurt, fresh seasonal fruit, and presoaked oil-rich seeds	sunflower oil
oatmeal and water	mashed banana or rasped apple	coconut oil, cinnamon
whole grain sourdough bread	omelet + vegetables	pepper, sea salt
whole wheat bread	preserves with no added sugar	unpasteurized butter
buckwheat pancakes	applesauce	cinnamon
quinoa	avocado, shrimp	rapeseed oil or olive oil, lemon
spelt bread with sunflower seeds	white-meat chicken or turkey	unpasteurized butter, olives, arugula, lettuce

TABLE 2 Breakfast as brainfood

If you have your last meal of the day at 8:00 pm and you don't eat again until noon the next day, you're telling your body to just figure it out for sixteen hours, while at the same time expecting optimal performance. A bit much to ask, don't you think? Have a breakfast full of macronutrients. Keep combinations in mind for the best results.

Your breakfast should be determined by what you had for dinner the evening before. If you had carbohydrates for dinner—pasta, rice or potatoes--have a protein-rich breakfast like an omelet with vegetables, a combination with quinoa or even a complete vegetable soup. Dare to start the day with a loaded vegetable omelet or even an avocado salad with shrimp. Avocado stimulates fat burning and since it's full of unsaturated fats, it's considered an essential fruit.

If you had no carbohydrates the evening before, have a breakfast that includes complex sugars like bran or rye bread. Bran includes the outer layer of the grain, making it rich in vitamins and minerals. Rye keeps your blood glucose levels constant and gives you a satisfied feeling. Combine your bread with unpasteurized butter or dip it in olive oil to add some fat. You can add jam to your sandwich or even vegetables like carrots, lettuce or pickles. My favorite breakfast is oatmeal cooked in water, along with mashed banana, coconut oil, and some honey for sweetness. Opt for unprocessed oats to get all the nutrients. Of course fruit is fine as well.

It's best to eat fruit on an empty stomach. A kiwi for breakfast prevents constipation and it's an excellent source of vitamin C. Yellow kiwi is best because it's less of a burden on your digestion. You could also have vegetable or fruit juice without added sugar. Freshly-made juices are excellent, especially when they include the pulp for fiber.

Avoid simple sugars like ready-made jam, Nutella, white bread, and the classic corn flakes. These elevate your blood glucose levels and give you a sugar dip later on.

Vitamins A, D, E, K, and essential fatty acids are dissolved by fats. So flavor your breakfast with unsaturated fats like nuts, pumpkin seeds, linseed, and avocadoes.

Training: Breakfast is essential in relation to morning training. Without breakfast your tank is only ¾ full, even if you ate well the day before. This is how it works: your body stores an excess of glucose as glycogen in your liver (25%), and in your muscles (75%). Since the energy stored in your liver the evening before is used for the nightly processes of your organs and brain, this store is all but gone by morning. Hence your ¾ full tank. If you ate little carbohydrate the evening before, your blood glucose is even lower. In the worst case your body has to get its energy from glycogenesis, which leads to muscle breakdown, energy loss, and acidification. We will explore all the details of this emergency process in Part Four.

If you absolutely don't have time for breakfast, at least try to have a hard-boiled egg, a granola bar, or a protein bar. If you feel that you really can't eat anything yet, at least have a thirst-quencher or a low-sugar beverage like Kombucha or a fruity iced tea.

Morning snack

Try to choose quality snacks whenever you can, like (dried) fruit and nuts or granola bars. Seasonal fruit is fine as well.

Lunch

Lunch gives you an extra boost. It prevents sleepiness and trouble concentrating at the end of the afternoon, but only if you opt for high-energy food. That means complex carbohydrates. Do eat enough, because if you don't, your blood glucose level will be low in the evening, and you'll crave sugar.

So, **complex carbohydrates prevent the afternoon energy dip**. Eat them with vegetables and not too much protein. Examples: dark bread with spring lettuce, or pasta with vegetable sauce, potatoes with vegetables, or rice with stirred vegetables. Soup, raw vegetables or salads are fine as well. The fiber in vegetables has a de-acidifying effect and keeps hunger at bay.

Legumes and grains with a low glycemic index also prevent hunger pangs later in the day. They, too, keep your blood glucose levels constant so you don't experience a sugar dip.

Avoid simple carbohydrates and heavy meals. They make you drowsy and increase your craving for sweets. If you do eat sweets, have them right after the meal or in combination with a protein. That way the impact on your blood glucose is lower than if you eat them on an empty stomach.

Afternoon snack

An afternoon snack tides you over until dinnertime. Without this snack, you run the risk of being famished by dinner time, and you might overeat. If you exercise after work, use the afternoon snack to get the necessary energy. Protein-rich foods like a protein bar, yogurt or a handful of almonds are all great choices. Vegetables (cooked or raw), vegetable juice, vegetable stock, or soup are fine as well.

Dinner

Dinner should be your lightest meal of the day. You don't want your meal to disturb your sleep, and anyway, you no longer need the energy. This is the moment to take in protein and lose the carbohydrates. Raw vegetables are a good alternative for processed starters.

Harder to digest proteins like **red meat or legumes aren't a good idea for dinner. Opt instead for easily digestible proteins like fish or poultry**. Limit your consumption--take it easy on the pasta, potatoes or bread. Rather, eat fish or chicken with vegetables, or a stir fry.

For a good night's rest, eat no later than two hours before going to bed. If you really want to have dessert or an evening snack around 10:00 pm, eat nuts, cheese or yogurt, but avoid coffee and simple sugars. A piece of dark chocolate (more than 70%) is fine too. It has polyphenols and antioxidants with infection-resistant qualities. The less sugar in the chocolate the better.

Beverages

Drink enough water. It's important for your entire body to stay hydrated, but especially for your brain. Dehydration immediately affects your performance. For instance, dry lips represent 2% dehydration and 10% loss of performance. Drinking gets fluids to your brain. A general guideline: drink 30 ml liquid/kg body weight a day.

Mineral water with sodium can contain more than 2 g salt per liter. Opt for mineral water with less than half an ounce of salt per liter, or filtered water.

Choose (red) wine over beer. Try to limit it to one glass with dinner. Strong liquors like vodka, brandy, or whiskey are best drunk on ice, without soda. Avoid sodas, and drink fruit juices only in the morning, on an empty stomach.

You can drink regular black coffee or espresso. Tea drinkers should opt for herbal or green tea. Leave out the sugar, though. If you like your beverages sweet, have fructose (fruit sugar) or—if you're on a low-calorie diet--opt for a sugar substitute like Stevia, which has zero calories and no negative side effects.

Dietary supplements

Dietary supplements are not meant to compensate for an unbalanced diet or lack of fluids. They can, however, promote physical and mental performance, and they can also contribute to recovery. So, to speed up recovery, by all means, take supplements.

There are two types of supplements:

- Primary dietary supplements (iron, vitamin B12, and folic acid) prevent anemia.
- Secondary dietary supplements support physical performance. This includes improving recovery.

In both cases, you should have a physical analysis or a blood test to determine which supplements you need. This ensures a good nutrient balance.

A good multivitamin can be taken without any tests, because it takes into account the interaction and ratio of vitamins and minerals. So the odds are small that your vitamin and mineral balances will be out of whack. Multivitamins help overall physical recovery and physical performance.

TAILORED NUTRITION PLAN

Food is energy, but it's all about the right amounts. Keeping your blood glucose levels constant is imperative. When you give your body a shot of simple sugars, you produce insulin to process the glucose. This leads to a sugar dip, which drains your energy and increases your craving for sweets.

When your blood glucose levels swing too often, you can become desensitized to insulin, and you end up in the risk group for type 2 diabetes. The extra-large supply of insulin also triggers the secretion of stress hormones, because suddenly your body has too much to handle. So what you eat affects your mood as well. Sugar dips, sugar cravings, type 2 diabetes, stress, mood swings--these are all issues you can do without. The following will help you create a nutrition plan tailored to your fatigue.

NUTRITION WHEN YOU'RE PHYSICALLY FATIGUED

General

Because adrenalin raises your blood glucose levels, you empty your tank without realizing it. The adrenalin gives you energy instead, but it's a false sense of fitness. Adrenalin sends the circulation to your muscles instead of to your digestion. Your inadequate digestion undermines your acid base balance, and a lack of stomach acid can make you feel bloated or give you acid reflux. Too much stomach acid can lead to flatulence.

Eat regularly and opt for light meals. Avoid simple sugars and combine proteins with carbohydrate to keep your blood glucose stable.

Breakfast

Have a protein-rich breakfast with soup, an omelet or vegetables. This way you get all the necessary nutrients without the sugar. If you do feel the need for carbohydrates, have some toast with fruit, or oatmeal with coconut oil. White bread, ripe bananas, jam, and chocolate are big no-nos. These simple sugars are stressors for your body. They raise your blood glucose sky high, which results in your feeling hungry. That's double stress! (Bananas in combination with oatmeal are an exception.)

Snacks

Eat a small meal every two hours, even when you're not hungry. Half an energy bar without added sugar or a sugar-free granola bar are good snacks. Eat berries in the summer--they're full of antioxidants. In the winter, eat apples, nectarines, and kiwi.

Lunch

Eat plenty of vegetables and some fish or white meat for lunch. Heavy meals with fat and protein feel like a brick in your stomach and might cause acid reflux.

Dinner
Eat protein and a complex carbohydrate after an evening recovery workout. Quinoa is ideal because it contains both.

You may not need any energy boosts in the morning because you get a fast start. But in the afternoon and in the evening, you may experience a dip. This means you're in overdrive, so avoid caffeine and other stimulants.

You need extra minerals such as sodium and potassium to counteract your elevated adrenalin levels. Adrenalin results in dehydration so drinking enough liquids is more important than ever.

NUTRITION WHEN YOU'RE HORMONALLY FATIGUED

General
If you're hormonally fatigued, the levels of the stress hormone cortisol determine your sense of hunger. If your cortisol levels are high, you might not feel hungry. However, don't wait to eat until you have a sugar dip, because then your body converts proteins to sugar, leading to elevated blood glucose. In addition to being an added stressor, this conversion from protein to glucose results in muscle degeneration. The big takeaway: timing is key.

Your inadequate digestion undermines your acid base balance, and the lack of stomach acid can make you feel bloated and gassy. Too much stomach acid can lead to acid reflux.

Breakfast
Have **breakfast at 10:00 am**. Your cortisol levels start rising at 6:00 am, with a peak at 8:00 am, so it's quite possible you're not hungry at that time. Don't give in to this feeling, though, because keeping your stomach empty causes a stress response. Your body worries because it's not getting any food. If you don't eat a big meal until 8:00 pm and your first meal the next day is at noon, you're depriving your body of quality nutrients for sixteen hours. In that case your body switches to survival mode to accommodate your energy needs.

Lunch
Anticipate your sugar dip. Have lunch early, between 11:30 am and 12:30 pm.

Afternoon snack
Have a nutritious snack (protein bar or granola bar) between 2:00 and 3:00 pm to prevent a cortisol dip.

Dinner
Have dinner around 6:00 to 7:00 pm.

Combine proteins with carbohydrates and fats. Eating only carbohydrates causes your blood sugar to rise too fast. Opt for complex carbohydrate, like brown rice, whole wheat, buckwheat, barley, whole oats, quinoa, etc. Eat as little refined sugar, white bread, or white pasta as possible.

Vegetables contain good carbohydrates, fiber, antioxidants, and minerals. Eat several servings of vegetables a day, in soup, green juice or steamed. Opt for leafy greens whenever possible. Especially seaweed and algae are chock-full of vitamins, minerals, and amino acids.

It's best to **take it easy on the fruit, because the high sugar content can cause your body extra stress**. Don't have your first fruit until around 10:15 am. Avoid bananas, raisins, dates, figs, and oranges, and have papaya, mango, plums, pears, kiwi, apples, cherries or melon instead. Combine your fruit with soy yogurt.

Increase your intake of iodine for optimal thyroid function. Your thyroid is underperforming as a result of your exhausted adrenal gland. Iodine—a trace element that can be found in bread and salt, but also in seaweed and wild fatty fish like sardines, anchovies, and salmon—aids the output of thyroid hormones. Fatty fish is also rich in omega-3 fatty acids, which regulate the thyroid hormone receptors. Include selenium, iron, zinc, and copper in your diet, too. These minerals are also essential for the output of thyroid hormones.

Use sea salt on your food. This sees to your craving for salt, and you need it to counteract your low blood pressure. Stay away from caffeine.

NUTRITION WHEN YOU'RE MENTALLY FATIGUED

General

Try to figure out why you're tired. Is there a concrete reason you have been performing in stress mode for a while? Has there been a compilation of stressful situations, with as a result trouble sleeping, feeling tired? Once this is clear, adjust your diet. If you have trouble sleeping, follow the tips for physical fatigue and use nutrition to positively affect your neurotransmitters. (More about these brain messengers in Chapter 15.) Since they have a big influence on your mood, appetite, rest, action, happiness, etc., it stands to reason that the function of your neurotransmitters determines how you feel.

Keep your blood glucose levels constant. Your brain doesn't burn fat--it only uses glucose as fuel, so it requires a constant blood glucose stream. If you have a low or strongly dropping blood glucose level, you become irritated, forgetful, you have mood swings, depression, trouble concentrating, etc. Make sure to eat before you're hungry and avoid simple sugars.

More than half of your brain's weight consists of fat. **Especially omega-3 fatty acids play a critical role** because they improve communication within your brain. Your body doesn't produce omega-3 fatty acids, so you get this mainly from fatty fish.

Consume plenty of vitamins and minerals. For you this is more important than ever. **Vitamins B1, B2, B6, folic acid, B12, and C** all contribute to forming, sending, and receiving neurotransmitters. Minerals like sodium, potassium, and calcium magnesium monitor the fluid balance and the brain's electric circuit. Know that a lack of just one nutrient can already have an effect on your neurotransmitters and your brain function.

NUTRITION WHEN YOU'RE METABOLICALLY FATIGUED

General

If you suffer from metabolic fatigue, your diet should be all about your biochemistry. This includes your acid base balance, mineral status, vitamins (such as B12, iron, and folic acid) and your intestinal flora. Extra vitamin B12, iron, and folic acid also help your aerobic energy system. Seek professional help to get a tailored diet based on your biochemical profile and discomforts.

A NOTE ON CAFFEINE

Caffeine can stimulate mental and physical activities. It indirectly causes the adrenal gland to produce adrenalin, which stimulates your central nervous system, heart rate, and blood pressure. It's best to avoid caffeine if you have trouble sleeping.

If, on the other hand, you need an extra energy boost now and then, a cup of coffee is fine, but you shouldn't make it a habit. Over time you become dependent, and then you need to drink more to get the same effect. This is a problem, because it's important to watch your portions. Low or medium doses of caffeine (100 – 175 mg) promote your focus and reduce the feeling of fatigue. Higher doses (more than 450 mg) will make you anxious, restless, and tense, and they dehydrate you. Too much caffeine can also lead to a slower uptake of minerals, and it can affect stomach acid production. The effect of the caffeine in coffee is nullified if you add sugar, because of the rise in your blood glucose levels.

Caffeine can be found in coffee, tea and cola:
- One cup of coffee (100 ml) = 70 mg caffeine
- One cup espresso (100 ml) = 170 mg caffeine
- One cup powder coffee (100 ml) = 56 mg caffeine
- One glass of coke (200 ml) = 20 mg caffeine
- One glass green tea (125 ml) = 30 mg caffeine

EATING OUT

If you have a lot of business lunches or if you just eat at restaurants a lot, you can still make healthy choices. Below are some tips for eating out.

Choice of restaurant
- Choose a Japanese or seafood restaurant when possible, and go for low-sodium soy sauce.
- Avoid fast food places.

Beverages
- Always have water at the beginning of a meal.
- If you want soda, opt for sugar free.
- Drink wine rather than beer, and preferably red wine. Limit yourself to two glasses of alcohol.

Appetizers
- It's better to have appetizers than dessert.
- Opt for soup or salad. Clear soups are better than the creamy kind.

Main course
- Choose fish over meat. If you do have meat, have white-meat poultry, not red meat like beef or pork.
- Opt for grilled or stir-fried dishes instead of fried.
- Take it easy on the potatoes, fries, rice, pasta, and bread.
- Choose brown rice, whole wheat bread, or quinoa.
- Choose leafy or brightly colored vegetables.
- Avoid high-fat creamy sauces. Have olive oil and lemon or a light dressing instead. Have some extra pepper if you must, but no extra salt.

Dessert
- Choose a savory dessert--like cheese--over a sweet one.
- Ask for your dessert without whipped cream or chocolate sauce.
- Ice cream is high in sugar, but it's coated by a layer of fat and protein from the milk. So its sugar enters your bloodstream

relatively slowly, without causing an overproduction of adrenalin. Even better is sugar free ice cream, sorbet or frozen yogurt.

- Coffee, mate and tea are fine, but without sugar or cookies. Stevia is a good sugar substitute. Erythritol is also a zero-calorie sugar substitute, but keep in mind that—unlike Stevia--it does affect your blood sugar levels.

CHAPTER 6:
TRAVEL

JET LAG

Travel is pretty intense for your body, because of the disruption of your biorhythm (and the bad food). The following explains how you can minimize the effects of jetlag. How you manage light is key. The trick is to adjust your starting biorhythm to your destination.

Travelling from east to west
Morning arrival: Avoid morning light. Wear sunglasses or a sleeping mask. Look for shady or dim places. Once you arrive at your destination, opt for a low-sugar breakfast with protein.

Evening arrival: expose yourself to as much light as possible to avoid wanting to go to sleep. At your destination, opt for sugars rather than protein.

Travelling from west to east
Morning arrival: set your rhythm earlier by stimulating your alertness. Get up earlier, take a shower, take a morning walk, or exercise to expose yourself to daylight. Continue exposing yourself to daylight as much as possible for the rest of the day. Avoid a nap--this can disrupt your sleep rhythm. Once you arrive at your destination, have protein for breakfast.

Evening arrival: don't expose yourself to intense light sources, or do intense exercise or work—you want to avoid stimulation. Swimming and sex are fine. At your destination, opt for complex carbohydrates and vegetables for dinner. These allow you to fall asleep easily. If you do eat protein, choose fish or poultry.

ALTITUDE TRAINING

Ten years ago, I spent three months in Switzerland to study the pros and cons of altitude training as an innovative training instrument for professional athletes. I found that the Swiss have centers where altitude training is not only provided for professional athletes, but also for executives. That's a good idea. Why? It saves time. A forty-minute workout at 1800 meters is the equivalent of a one-hour workout at sea level!

Two types of altitude training:
With **active altitude training**, you train wearing an oxygen-reducing mask, simulating altitude. This leads to better aerobic capacity, so your body uses energy more efficiently and you don't run on empty quite as soon. By doing focused altitude training, professional athletes can experience an increase in the duration of maximum performance. Because your anaerobic threshold is lower at altitude, your VO2max--or your maximum oxygen uptake per kg body weight--also drops. If your VO2max is 160 at sea level, it can be 145 at an altitude of 1800 meters. In order to get the desired effect, it's crucial to correctly determine your VO2max at the start of your training program. If you end up running on empty, all the positive effects are gone. The average duration of this workout is forty minutes.

With **passive altitude training**, you focus on brake performance and reducing your empathetic activities. (More on this in Chapter 15.) This promotes recovery capacity, so stress has less of an impact on your body. You do this by, for instance, sitting for five minutes with the mask and five minutes without. The total duration varies from thirty to sixty minutes.

For optimal effect it's best to sustain your altitude training for three to twelve weeks, with an average of two to three sessions a week, based on a plan tailored to your needs. I recommend you get your blood tested for anemia at the start of such a training program. Checking the blood oxygen levels during the training program is also important. The oxygen saturation is usually 98%, but during altitude training this can drop to 70%. For good results it's crucial to check your oxygen saturation and heart rate at each step.

Altitude training is also a good preparation for cycling events like scaling Mont Ventoux (France) or climbing Mount Everest.

CHAPTER 7:
MENTAL RELAXATION

Mental relaxation means inserting a rest period, so your batteries can get fully recharged, and you're in control of your own thoughts and schedule again. It also means being in a safe, comforting environment.

FROM EXERTION TO RELAXATION

Mental relaxation is quite personal. What's relaxing for one might be an exertion for another. Some people enjoy an evening out with friends while others would rather spend their free time alone. For some, cooking or gardening clears the head--others consider these to be chores. So you have to determine for yourself what relaxes you. You have so many responsibilities, so many others to answer to. Be mindful that your relaxation doesn't end up becoming yet another obligation.

Relaxing activities, are activities you truly feel like doing and that you yourself choose to do. Going out for dinner, listening to music, exercising, visiting an art gallery, or simply hanging out at home—anything goes, as long as it gives you a good feeling. Once you know what relaxes you, don't hesitate to insert this activity into your schedule at regular times. Here's an example of some ways to insert rest periods:

- Every hour: short breaks like you had back in school. One ten-minute break for every fifty minutes of work (bathroom break, drinking, eating)
- Every day: thirty minutes for yourself
- Per week: half a day for yourself
- Per month: a weekend
- Per year: a vacation

Be selfish. It's appropriate in this case. By doing this, you protect yourself and everyone you care about from your stress. And it's good for your health.

GOOD RELATIONSHIPS FOR GOOD HEALTH

Being valued by others and having a sense of self-worth provide a strong, balanced foundation, and love and warmth are vital aids. Both give you an overall sense of rest and recovery. Human relationships are essential, therefore, as long as they make you feel comfortable and safe. Communication, trust, openness, honesty, and respect are the building blocks for any good relationship. Good relationships give you confidence, they make you feel loved, and they give you a more positive outlook. In short, good relationships have a direct impact on your health. The opposite is also true--a relationship with someone you trust is pleasant, while dealing with someone you don't trust is exhausting.

Cuddling and sex are also good for your health. Cuddling reduces blood pressure and it gets the pleasure hormones streaming through your body. Caressing the skin can even make you shudder and give you goosebumps.

Regular sex contributes to your overall physical well-being, strengthens your immune function, and increases your life expectancy. Sex has a big effect on stress, because sexual arousal spurs the release endorphins, the feel-good hormones. It even has a painkilling effect, which you experience as relaxation and complete release. So, ladies, there's a reason men usually fall asleep like a log after having sex! Also, you use as many calories during sex as during swimming--200 to 300 calories in thirty minutes, so you can even consider it a recovery workout.

MASSAGES

A massage has a local and recovering effect on the body through direct contact with the skin and indirect contact with the muscles. Massages are also addictive. Once you've had one, you'll want to have one more often.

Two types of massage:

• If you have stiff muscles—neck and back pain, for instance--as the result of acute stress responses, have a relaxing massage to get rid of the muscle tension. Too intense and direct contact with the skin or muscles can lead to yet another stress response. The main thing here is to relax the muscles.
• If you feel lethargic, it's better to have a stimulating massage. This increases muscle tension and gives your body an energy boost.

When you have your first ever massage, make it a relaxing one and wait to see how your body responds. If you're used to massages, your body can take more and it won't respond acutely to the stress stimulus.

TAILORED RELAXATION PLAN

Mental relaxation is the fourth building block of good health—everyone needs it. Take the time for it, even when you don't feel it's a priority. It's an important component of recovery, so adjust your expectations and set more realistic goals if that's what it takes to insert it into your schedule.

Relaxation when you're physically fatigued

You set the bar too high. The gap between your mental wishes and your physical limits is too big. The adrenalin makes you impatient, short-fused, and puts you in fight mode. You're quick to feel attacked. You tend to react more emotionally than you used to, and in general you don't feel like your normal self. Over time you lose focus and concentration. There's a danger that you'll say things you'll regret, and which you'll have to answer for later on. This sometimes happens in frustration, because your mind wants to move forward, but your body steps on the brakes. The right physical capacity can prevent lots of trouble.

- Set realistic goals and adjust your expectations.
- Work per the school system. Insert little breaks--five to ten minutes--every fifty minutes. Stretch your legs, go chat with a coworker, or have a snack outside. These little breaks allow you to catch your breath and to calm down from the adrenalin rush of the moment.
- Do three fun things a day. You can do them by yourself or with the people you love.
- Drink plenty of water and eat snacks. This supports your central nervous system with the necessary fluids and energy, so you're less short-fused.
- Meditation is a life saver for some people. It allows you to reconnect with your whole body.

Relaxation when you're hormonally fatigued

When you're chronically fatigued, you may feel lethargic, drowsy and apathetic. The fatigue can even affect your personality. At heart, you may be action-oriented, but your chronic fatigue makes you procrastinate at tasks. You're chronically tired and your expectations are not in line with what you can handle. The emotional impulse has an impact on your adrenal glands. Take, for instance, the death of a loved one or problems at work. But positive emotions like the birth of a child or marriage also have pitfalls. They're fine things to look forward to, but they're still stressors.

- Get informed. Find out what's wrong with you--figure out the real cause of your symptoms. Not knowing leads to worry and doubt.
- Set realistic goals and adjust your expectations.
- Dare to make decisions according to how you think and feel about the matter in question.
- Do three fun things a day. You can do them alone or with loved ones if you want.

Relaxation when you're mentally fatigued

Emotions tend to have an impact on your adrenal glands, so you feel less energetic. An action plan might be appropriate for you. This will help you

77

find more mental rest, and you don't need to ask yourself all the time whether you're doing the right thing.

- Determine how you think about things, both emotionally and rationally. Stand up for yourself and your choices.
- Don't feel guilty - take care of yourself. Only when you feel good and you have control over your emotions, can you make others happy.
- Work according to the school system. Insert a little break--five to ten minutes--every fifty minutes. Stretch your legs, chat with a coworker or eat a snack outside. This is good for your focus and your mental battery. Include these little breaks when you plan your day.

Relaxation when you're metabolically fatigued

Perhaps you've been working out intensely on willpower alone, or perhaps something else is exhausting you. Either way, your fuel tank is empty. You must take good care of yourself and treat your body with mindfulness. If not, you'll feel tired and sluggish in the evening.

You don't want to set yourself up for failure. With a good understanding of your fatigue, you'll be able to set realistic goals for your body.

Prepare yourself nutritionally for your physical exertions during the day. Have a high-energy meal before an evening workout. It prevents your tank from running out of fuel.

CHAPTER 8:
SLEEP

Many patients tell me they have trouble falling asleep, they wake up during the night, they wake up in the morning feeling drowsy, or they feel tired during the day. Sleeping pills can give temporary relief, but I would advise strongly against prolonged use. Addiction, drowsiness or reduced alertness in traffic can be side effects. It's better to listen to your body and anticipate any trouble sleeping.

Adrenalin and cortisol keep you awake if you suffer from physical or hormonal fatigue, or you worry about numerous issues if you suffer from mental fatigue. That makes sense, because you work hard and you don't know when to stop.

Your trouble with sleep is often the result of a deeper problem, namely the body's reduced capacity to recover.

This chapter explains the benefits of sleep, helps you understand your own sleep, and offers solutions.

SLEEP: YOUR BODY'S MAINTENANCE

Adequate sleep at night is essential for both your mental and physical health.

Mental health: First of all, getting enough sleep has several benefits for your memory and cognitive processes. When you sleep, you transfer information from your short-term memory to your long-term memory. That's how you are able to learn while you sleep.

Sleep is also a kind of car wash for your brain. The many mental processes in the analytical and emotional area of your brain create neurotoxins and waste protein. A good night's rest takes care of eliminating these waste products, which have been linked to dementia, among other things.

Physical health: Sleep plays a vital role in general physical recovery. Your muscles and body recover from exertions and fatigue while you sleep. Your body produces growth hormones as you sleep, which allow for cell regeneration. Sleep also stimulates the formation of antibodies, so your immune function gets a boost.

When you don't get enough sleep, your body produces the stress hormone cortisol, which works against your immune function. Several other hormonal changes also occur with a lack of sleep, such as the production of hormones that stimulate your appetite, and especially your sweet tooth. When you have too much of a sweet tooth, you become insensitive to insulin. This is why, a lack of sleep also increases your risk of type 2 diabetes.

THE STRUCTURE OF SLEEP

Nowadays most people in the industrialized countries go through four to five ninety-minute sleep cycles a night, each consisting of five stages. Yet this classic sleeping pattern is less classic or universal than you'd think. Let's go back in time before we discuss the different stages.

Past and Present
Before the discovery of electricity, the human sleeping pattern consisted of about twelve hours, but with a break, according to historian Robert Ekirch. 'First sleep' began around dusk and lasted four or five hours. Following that, people were awake for two or three hours. This intermission was ideal for reading, praying, visiting friends, or making love. Then they would go to sleep again until morning. The introduction of electric light, at the end of the nineteenth century, threw a wrench in that natural rhythm--people were happy to have the extra productive time.

Although first and second sleep may seem strange concepts now, studies show that this is still our natural rhythm. Experiments by psychiatrist

Thomas Wehr have shown that, without artificial light, we don't stay awake for sixteen hours, but rather for barely ten. Though his test subjects initially slept all the way through, over time they adopted a similar rhythm as that of our ancestors: they slept for four or five hours, were awake for a few hours, and then slept till morning. In places without artificial light, people still have this rhythm. This paleo rhythm tells us it's quite normal to wake up in the middle of the night. It's also quite normal to not sleep deeply. After all, for our ancestors, sleeping through noise could be fatal.

THE CIRCADIAN RHYTHM

We all know the term 'biorhythm'. We tend to call ourselves either morning or evening people. But did you know that your nervous system, hormones, muscles, and organs—in short, all your biological functions—follow a preprogrammed day rhythm? It's a result of the evolution of our species. This is what it looks like:

• Between 5:00 and 8:00 am: the active stage—you're alert, energetic, and you have a better short-term memory.
• Between 11:00 am and 2:00 pm: a stage of weaker physical performance—you're introverted and tired.
• Between 5:00 and 8:00 pm: a new stage of increased alertness and physical readiness.
• Between 11:00 pm and 2:00 am: a stage of fatigue and little alertness.
• Between 2:00 am and 5:00 am: the weakest stage.

When you function according to these stages, you function according to your internal clock. Of course, external disturbances like jet lags, fatigue, and night shifts can also cause you to run behind or ahead of schedule.

The five stages of sleep

Our sleep consists of five ninety-minute cycles. Some research speaks of four cycles. You wake up briefly at the end of every cycle, even though you may not be aware of it. These ninety-minute cycles consist of several stages:

- **Stage 0:** before falling asleep--several seconds to ten minutes. Your muscles are still tense and you have rapid eye movements. You experience every sound or thought as distracting.
- **Stage 1:** falling asleep--one to seven minutes. You hover in between consciousness and sleep. Your respiration and heart rate slow down. You may experience muscle shocks.
- **Stage 2:** slow sleep--10 to 25 minutes. Your eye movements slow down. You're less aware your surroundings, though loud noises may still wake you. Your temperature drops.
- **Stage 3:** transition to deep sleep--a few minutes. Your brain activity and muscles relax. You fall into deep sleep.
- **Stage 4:** deep sleep or recovery stage--twenty to forty minutes. In this stage your body recovers--your fuel tank is refilled. Your blood pressure drops, your respiration slows even more, your muscles are now fully relaxed and get more blood, your body produces growth hormones so muscles, tissue and bones can heal.
- **Stage 5:** REM sleep (Rapid Eye Movement)--one to five minutes. In this stage you are still fast asleep. You notice little of noises in your surroundings, your muscles are switched off, but your eyes make rapid movements, and your breathing quickens. Your brain is also active--you dream and process information. Men sometimes get an erection during this stage.

Because each cycle lasts ninety minutes, it's best to work with ninety-minute blocks when setting your alarm clock. That way you're more likely to wake up at the end of a cycle, rather than interrupting one halfway through. Seven and a half hours of sleep is a good average, but depending on your needs, this can be ninety minutes more or less. Even when you don't go to bed until 1:00 am, it's better to sleep for 4.5 hours than for five. If you're fatigued, it's obviously better to sleep longer.

SLEEP AND HORMONES

Your cortisol levels start to rise around 6:00 am, washing away your sleep hormone melatonin, so you have the energy to start your day. Your cortisol continues to rise until around noon--then it diminishes. Stress can disrupt this pattern, however. High cortisol levels in the evening make you feel energetic, so you go to bed late. Your sleep pattern is disturbed and the growth hormone—which is responsible for your recovery—is less effective. Low cortisol levels in the morning make you drowsy and it takes you a while to get started.

With our lifestyle, we tend to ignore the sleep hormone melatonin, which is sensitive to light. Nature has programmed us so we produce melatonin when it gets dark. That's what makes you feel sleepy in the evening. We can disturb this mechanism in two ways: with cortisol and with artificial light, especially blue screens like smart phones, laptops etc. These keep your serotonin levels high. In both cases you don't feel the need to sleep.

Of course, nutrition plays a role in relation to your sleep. It's also related to your hormones:

- Milk indirectly stimulates melatonin production.
- Caffeinated beverages (coffee, tea, cola, etc.) decrease the production of melatonin.
- Simple carbohydrates slow down the supply of growth hormones because they spur insulin production, the opposite of your growth hormone.

LIGHT

Make sure you get enough daylight every day. Go outside for fifteen minutes during your lunch break. Even when it's overcast there's still enough daylight to feel the positive effects, like the production of vitamin D. Cycling or walking to work in the morning allows you to get a good shot of daylight so your biorhythm is adjusted.

Artificial light: intensity

If you spend a lot of time in an office, the quality of the lighting is important. Unfortunately, the only thing we tend to require of lighting is that it allows us to see well. We seldom pay much attention to the light intensity. Outside, this ranges from 10,000 to 20,000 lux on a sunny day and 1,000 lux when it's overcast, while inside it's barely 500 lux. To mimic the intensity of natural light, you can increase the intensity of artificial light to 800 lux.

Artificial light: color
• Even more important than the intensity is the light's color:
• White-blue light stops the secretion of your sleep hormone melatonin. It makes you active and clear-headed. It stimulates you, so it's ideal for feeling fit during the day;
• Yellow-blue light also suppresses melatonin production;
• Red light spurs the production of melatonin. It's warm, cozy and relaxing.

TIPS FOR A GOOD NIGHT'S REST

A good night's rest begins with good preparation. Here are some general tips to help get you started:

- You spend about a third of your life in bed, so invest in a good one.
- Avoid consumption of sweet, processed food and stimulants after 4:00 pm. For instance, no coffee, tobacco, chocolate, sugar or meat.
- Create a ritual about thirty minutes before bed that tells your brain it's soon time to sleep. Your brain will send your body the necessary signals.
- Don't do any cognitive or physical activities thirty minutes before bed. Swimming, recovery training, and sex are allowed, but other activities are best done during the day. A bath also has a calming effect, as opposed to a shower.
- Make sure the bedroom is dark. If you have the lights on, your body thinks it's still day. Use your bedroom for its intended purpose: sleeping and sex. That means no television, no computers in bed, and no books on your night stand. Avoid all blue light, including digital alarm clocks.
- Keep your bedroom cool. The lower temperature helps you fall asleep. Use an extra blanket if you have to. Note that digestion and spicy food can raise your temperature, but these can easily be avoided.

- Get up if you wake up in the middle of the night. Like our ancestors, you should do something relaxing in between first and second sleep, and then go back to bed. Avoid bright light. Eating is also not a good idea.
- Train your internal clock: go to bed and rise at the same times as much as possible, even on weekends.

TAKE AN AFTERNOON NAP

People in warm countries around the Mediterranean Sea and in Central and South America take siestas. This way they avoid the hottest time of day, and they break the circadian rhythm--which covers a day--in two.

I would like us Belgians, in our colder climate, to have siestas as well. It's a rest period for the body, so it can put the brakes on your stress hormone and recover. Studies show that a nap doesn't mess up your nightly sleeping pattern. On the contrary, both types of sleep complement each other and contribute to good health. The benefits for your heart are tremendous. A Greek study shows that working men who regularly take an afternoon nap have about three times less chance of dying a premature coronary death.

These are the major benefits of a nap:
- Less fatigue because of the restorative effect
- Recovery, alertness, and focus
- Increase of your cognitive abilities (memory, learning, and information retrieval)
- A healthy heart, because you chase away your stress

An effective afternoon nap doesn't have to be long--between 15 and 45 minutes is enough. When we speak of a power nap or a micro nap, we mean moments of rest that take from a few to at most ten minutes--in the best case it increases your alertness for the next ten minutes. Micro naps of thirty to ninety seconds have no effect at all.

TAILORED SLEEP PLAN

We sleep ninety minutes less today than we did fifty years ago. We live in a society where we communicate 24/7 across different time zones. Sometimes sleep feels like a waste of time. But respecting your sleep is still fundamental to your general health. Break that rule and the punishment is immediate. Of course, everyone is different. It's possible to temporarily do with less sleep, but there's no such person as Superman or Superwoman. Even the most powerful people on earth need to sleep. That goes for you, too, even if you don't feel tired. The following provides tips tailored to your fatigue.

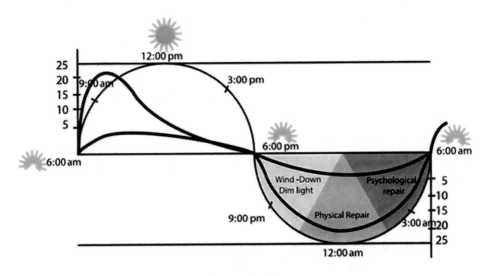

Cortisol level during day and night
IMAGE 4 Your cortisol and melatonin levels during day and night

Sleep when you're physically fatigued

- Your adrenalin frequently gets you out of bed early—sometimes even at 4:00 or 5:00 am—and by mid-afternoon you've done massive amounts of work. Take regular breaks. They can counter your (false) sense of energy, allowing you to get in touch with your body.
- Take a 15 - 45-minute nap in the afternoon. Your high adrenalin levels tell you that you don't need a nap, but it will definitely benefit you. A nap gives your body a rest signal, which allows your adrenalin to drop.

- If actual sleep is hard, do a brief meditation. Close your eyes, focus on your body, and make a mental body scan. This allows you to empty your mind for a moment while you receive the signs your body gives off.
- Spend at least half an hour outside during the day. Daylight indirectly results in an increased production of your sleep hormones. Even if it's overcast, you still get enough UV rays to have this benefit. Artificial light, and especially blue light, on the other hand, disturbs the production of melatonin.
- Prepare for your night's sleep. You might have a hard time falling asleep at night. Around 7:00 pm you crash in your easy chair, but falling asleep a few hours later is a major challenge. In that case, take a warm bath or a short recovery walk before you go to bed. Focus on your body and your breathing--three counts in and five counts out.
- If your sleep at night is regularly disturbed, focus even more on recovery training and/or resting moments during the day. Take a nap or do some meditation.

Sleep when you're hormonally fatigued

Your low cortisol levels make it hard for you to get up in the morning. Snoozing is your daily habit and even then, it's a challenge to get out of bed. More sleep at night and going to bed on time are more than ever essential.

- Go to bed around 10:00 pm and try not to stay awake past 10:30. If you stay awake later, your adrenal glands work overtime.
- On the weekend, give yourself some extra sleep, to 7:00 to 9:00 am. This relieves your adrenal glands.
- Forcing yourself and exhausting yourself is not recommended. On the other hand, don't feel sorry for yourself—maintain some discipline.

Sleep when you're mentally fatigued

Since your brain is in overdrive, it might be hard for you to fall asleep, and you get stuck in a downward spiral. Break it by preparing for sleep with relaxing evening activities and the proper breathing technique.

- Watch your breathing. At about one kilo, your brain weighs only a fraction of your total body weight. However, this energy hog does require 15 to 20% of your blood. Only if you breathe through your belly in the right rhythm (three counts in, five counts out) does your brain get constant circulation, and therefore the essential oxygen and energy.
- A recovery workout is the ideal segue from mental activities to sleep. Take an evening walk if you can't fall asleep, even if you were already in bed. You can also make this walk a standard component of your evening routine.
- Don't expose yourself to artificial light, including blue light from television or computer screens. The light keeps you awake and disturbs the production of melatonin.

Sleep when you're metabolically fatigued

When you're metabolically fatigued, falling asleep usually isn't a problem. But do ask yourself why you wake up in the middle of the night. Is it hunger, or does a stressor pump up your adrenalin? Remember, Metabolic fatigue goes hand in hand with other forms of fatigue.

LET'S RECAP

1. **Food is energy**. Stay one step ahead of feeling hungry. Plan your meals and use eating as a recovery moment for your body.

2. If you want to feel more energetic during the day, have breakfast like a king, lunch like a prince, and dine like a beggar. **It's best to eat six times a day**--three main meals and three snacks.

3. **The glycemic index** is the number that indicates the impact of the food on your blood glucose levels. The lower the glycemic index of a food is, the more stable your blood glucose remains.

4. **Complex carbohydrates** like whole-grain bread and whole-grain pasta, oatmeal, or brown rice have a low glycemic index. Their fiber minimizes blood glucose spikes and make you feel satisfied.

5. **Simple carbohydrates** have a high glycemic index. They cause spikes and drops in your blood glucose levels. As a result, you develop an increased craving for sweets.

6. **Mental relaxation** means inserting a rest period now and then, so your batteries can get fully recharged. Take the time for it, even when you don't feel it's a priority. By doing so, you protect yourself and everyone you care about from your stress.

7. A lot of body maintenance takes place while you **sleep**. The mental processes in your brain create neurotoxins and waste protein. A good night's rest takes care of eliminating them.

8. **While you sleep**, your muscles and body recover from exertions and fatigue. Growth hormones are produced as you sleep, which allow for cell regeneration. Sleep stimulates the formation of antibodies, so your immune function gets a boost.

9. Our sleep consists of **five ninety-minute cycles**, which in turn consist of several stages. Because each cycle lasts ninety minutes, it's best to work with ninety-minute blocks when setting your alarm clock. By doing so, you have a smaller chance of a rude awakening halfway a cycle.

10. **Take a nap** every now and then. It's a rest period for the body, so it can put the brakes on your stress hormone and recover.

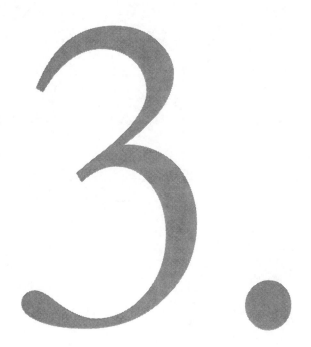

RECLAIM YOUR BODY

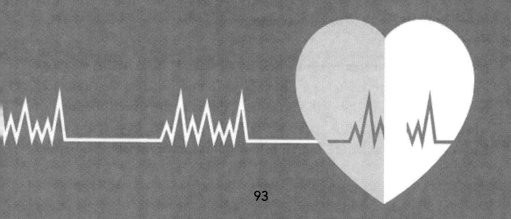

CHAPTER 9:
PHYSICAL SOLUTIONS FOR YOUR FATIGUE

Thanks to the adrenalin released during a workout, you may feel as if exercise gives you energy after a draining day at the office. As we have seen, though, this is deceptive, because your body can't tell the difference between stress at work, or in your private life, or stress from working out. You might feel a mental boost, but for your body the effects are the same. Working out when you're exhausted puts an even heavier burden on your already tired body.

Be aware of your fatigue. Accept it--don't settle for thinking fatigue is a luxury problem, because fatigue can definitely make you sick. No doubt coffee, badly scheduled workouts and some willpower can help you to function at your present level for another few months or even years, but you're not reaching your full potential and your fatigue will just accumulate.

What follows are some general guidelines to give you an idea of what you can expect when you start or get back into exercise and training when you're fatigued. In reality I advise each individual to work on a holistic action plan so nothing is left to chance. After all, one type of fatigue often affects another, so a tailored approach is best.

BASIC MOBILITY

Mobility is the first step toward a healthy lifestyle. Unfortunately, we move less and less in this digital age. Humans were built to cross vast distances on the savanna, and doing the occasional sprint in the search for food or when danger lurked. But today we take the car. Our biggest threat no longer comes from nature but from our (work) environment. You spend most of your time sitting in your office or in your car. If you make long days, you're sedentary for up to ten hours at a time. When you come home, you unwind in front of the TV or with a book or at a nice restaurant, adding even more sedentary time.

But sitting is going backward. Just like smoking, hypertension, and heart disease, sitting is a risk factor for your health. The evidence can be found in countless studies, and the World Health Organization (WHO) agrees. We have traded our endurance and vitality for Western diseases.

When you use your heart muscle less, the heart weakens, pumping less blood and oxygen to your organs. Because of your reduced basic endurance, you tend to switch to the anaerobic system (more on that in Part Four). Over time this can lead to heart complaints. If you add to that the fight-or-flight response as a result of a stressor, you accelerate the process. Theoretically, you can reach a heart rate of 250 beats per minute (which happens with some heart irregularities), but your body doesn't allow this under normal circumstances. It produces lactic acid, which stiffens your muscles. This is a natural brake on physical exertion.

A sedentary lifestyle also results in a reduced recovery capacity—indirectly, you become more susceptible to bacteria and viruses. Your biological processes don't work the way they should, and you're on your way to premature aging. So, moving is a basic need. It provides much-needed relaxation, and it keeps your muscles and joints supple. This is why, specialists recommend getting up and stretching your legs every thirty minutes, and actually moving at least thirty minutes per day. This can include walking stairs, gardening, walking, or parking the car further from your destination.

Looking ahead to your later years, moving gives you a lower risk of chronic disease, depression, physical limitations, and dementia. In return you have a more rewarding social life. You can live happily and independently for much longer.

But basic mobility doesn't suffice. Mobility helps sustain your health, but it doesn't lead to the recovery of a fatigued body or recovery after an intense performance. It doesn't help you lose weight, either. In short, basic mobility is essential, but you need more to reach your potential.

EXERCISE

Exercise is a broad term. It includes such wide-ranging activities as walking, playing ball, cross training, ultra-walking, skydiving, or climbing Mount Everest without oxygen tanks. A recent trend is that everything needs be longer, more intense, faster, and more challenging. Otherwise you don't count. Events like a 20K through Brussels are fully booked in no time. Finishing a quarter triathlon is no longer sexy enough. No, we all join in Iron Man and other excessive events. The question is, at what price? Especially considering that exercise is the only burden on your body you have complete control over, I sometimes wonder about the way people treat their bodies.

Since exercise stressors are equal to any other stressor, I'm not surprised at the waiting lists for sleep clinics, and that many people end up suffering burnout. I don't mean to scare you away from sports. Quite the contrary, those who approach it correctly reap the rewards. But it's important to consider that you run a marathon mostly to stroke your ego. That would be just fine, were it not that many never reach the finish line because they trained incorrectly. It's equally disturbing that many people can't manage a 5k after training for ten weeks. They quit after a few weeks, due injuries or other discomfort. So, you have to wonder: is physical exercise healthy or damaging to the body?

CAN PHYSICAL EXERCISE DAMAGE YOUR HEALTH?

Physical exercise can result in injuries, often due to lack of preparation and knowledge of both the body and training. Consider, for instance, the importance of a warmup, stretching, proper hydration, recovery, diet, as well as the importance of dietary supplements, good running shoes, technique, etc. The more intensely you exercise, the more you risk minor discomfort or injury, from tendonitis to joint wear and tear caused by dehydration. If you're addicted to exercise, you may find it hard to rest until an injury is completely healed. Overdoing it is the norm for hard-core exercisers.

A professional athlete's career lasts an average of fifteen years. Top performance demands a lot, and many professional athletes have about ten times more risk for arthritis once their career is over than the average person. That's just one of the many things top sport does to the human body. On the other hand, a professional athlete can count on a team of specialists, including kinetic therapists, personal trainers, mental coaches and dietitians. They get the necessary support, which helps to keep their risk of injury as low as possible. They also prepare for their physical performance with a well-thought-out training schedule. That's the difference between professional and amateur sports.

I can't overstate the value of a good training program. So many of us just do whatever, without giving much thought to the extreme performance and conditions we expose our body to. We work out without a proper schedule and we ignore the need for rest and recovery. We settle for a cheap gym membership, or information from the Internet, or we gather tips here and there, thinking we can avoid spending money on the right guidance. A good personal trainer is expensive, to be sure, but so is the price you pay if your body slowly deteriorates.

If you don't know enough about nutrition, oxidative stress raises its ugly head. (More about oxidative stress in Chapter 16.) So, it won't surprise you that few injuries are pure. By this I mean that most injuries aren't the result of exercise, but of infections resulting from fatigue. In some cases, showing up unprepared for an event can even have fatal consequences. We have no precise statistics, but it's been estimated that in Belgium, 100 to 200 people die every year of heart failure while exercising. The culprit is often a congenital abnormality, so it's not an unnecessary luxury to get a medical exam and a proper training schedule.

RELAXATION, NOT EXERTION

Maybe you are one of those people who go straight to the gym for an intense workout after a stressful day at the office. It clears the mind, supposedly. Unfortunately, this is only an added assault on your body. When you give an already fatigued body even more stressors, in the long run you inevitably suffer from exhaustion, burnout, depression, etc.

Fighting mental stress with physical stress will do you in. When you go running after an exhausting day at work, you exhaust your adrenal gland and use up your last reserves. Over time your resilience suffers and your immune function weakens. Heavy physical exertion both at work and in your free time actually leads to an increased risk of heart disease. (For other symptoms, see Chapter 2.) The message is loud and clear: you need relaxation after stress, not intense exertion. Exercise like walking and swimming are fine--light to medium exercise reduces your stress hormone levels.

Watching sports can be dangerous as well, because supporters are subject to stress. Since the rising adrenalin levels aren't accompanied by any physical exertion to justify your rapid heartbeat, being in the stands can be lethal. Also, supporters tend to reach for alcohol, tobacco, and high-fat foods to compensate for their lack of action. At the height of the game, the supporter crashes, because his cardiovascular system fails. The result: hypertension, trouble breathing, irregular heartbeat, heart attack, heart failure, etc. So, inertia can also cause damage.

CHAPTER 10:
TRAINING POSSIBILITES

Many people confuse exercise with training. Unlike with exercise, where it's more about the instant gratification and short-term stimuli, training is a long-term, comprehensive process. Training is carried out according to the laws of training science and exertion physiology. An individual program, tailored to your needs, is based on certain heart rate zones and aimed at reaching specific goals. It is this comprehensive process that allows you to exercise safely, with a fit body. You must be well-rested—it's a vital condition. A fatigued body isn't trainable and shouldn't be burdened.

This is the problem with all the books on training. They all assume your body is rested and that therefore it can be burdened. That is a huge mistake. Having fifteen years of experience as a physician, I can say with confidence that seven in ten people are fatigued, and incapable of following a training program without risk of injury. Starting with recovery training allows the body to rest and prevents injuries.

The important take-away is that it's not your fitness level that determines if you can train, but your level of fatigue. If you're like most people, physical fitness isn't the starting point for training. Your form is, and that includes your fatigue.

YOUR FITNESS PARAMETER

You can easily determine your fitness parameter with an exertion test. Your fitness parameter is your VO2max--or your maximum oxygen uptake/kg body weight. Therefore, the fastest way to enhance your fitness is to lose weight. This parameter is relatively constant in people who aren't professional athletes, because it doesn't fluctuate daily. After all, when you prepare for a competition, this parameter can increase. Form is different, because your fatigue *can* change daily. This is why it's crucial to consider form at the start of each training process. This process consists of two major phases: training toward a goal and training as a means to improve your health.

TRAINING TOWARD A GOAL OR AS A MEANS TO IMPROVE YOUR HEALTH

Training (or exercise) is the one stressor you control completely. Tiring out the body through interval training or any other type of exercise is only recommended for a rested body. When you're not fully recovered from previous stressors and you have no rest in your private and/or work life, you must do recovery training first. Your level of fatigue should determine the choice between training as a means to improve your health and training toward a goal. Since exercise is a vital part of your road to good health, this choice is crucial.

If you're not interested in exercise, it's still worthwhile to train as a means to improve your health. Consider training as a basic need, like sleep and nutrition. Your health and your performance at work and in your private life will benefit from recovery training, even if you have no athletic ambitions. It increases your body's ability to recover, and as a result you don't get tired as quickly. That pays off in the long run. If, five to ten years from now, you want to be able to burden your body to the same extent as you do today, this training program is vital.

RECOVERY: TRAINING AS A MEANS TO IMPROVE YOUR HEALTH

Recovery training is the best way to approach physical fatigue. It enables your body to tolerate more, and it will take you longer to reach your limits. After all, your physical performance not only depends on your endurance, but also on your body being well-rested. Even if you've never had any condition training, your performance will improve with recovery training. Let me illustrate what fatigue does to you. As a modestly competitive cyclist I will never be able to reach Tom Boonen's top speed. However, if I take him on after he has just finished the Tour of Flanders, I might stand a chance. The reason is simple: Tom's body is tired and I'm well-rested, despite the fact that Tom's condition is still better than mine. So you benefit tremendously from first investing in a well-rested body.

Recovery training consists of two phases:
The first phase results in a rested body. The length of this phase depends on your capacity (personal situation, family and work) and the level of your fatigue. Your body's stress response to training stimulates all vital functions—heart rate, muscle tension, and blood glucose. But if you don't exercise much, your body does little with these increases. On the contrary, you may experience burn-in. Recovery training gives a purpose to your increased blood glucose, muscle tension, and heart rate. As a result, your capacity increases and you have less risk of developing typically Western diseases like high blood pressure, heart disease, back and neck pain, metabolic syndrome, and diabetes. Walking, swimming, and cycling are all examples of recovery training.

Remember, recovery training—like any exercise—always has to be well-thought-out, and focused on a certain duration in a certain heart zone. Only then do you provide an efficient, targeted release for your body's stress responses. You should do recovery training mostly in the evening, for an average of fifteen minutes.

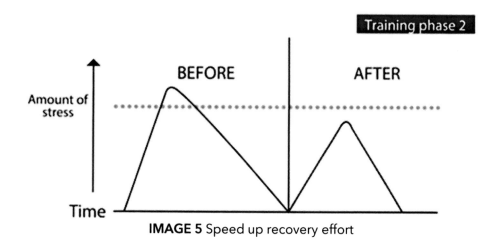

IMAGE 5 Speed up recovery effort

The second phase develops your body's ability to recover. A better brake system results in fewer high stress peaks as well as a faster recovery from stress. That's why I advise everyone who values their health not to skip this phase. It helps you to last longer and recover more quickly from fatigue. Your cardiac output--the amount of blood your heart pumps per minute—improves, and your resting heartbeat drops. Example: Experienced endurance athletes have a sleeping heart rate of barely 28 to 30 beats per minute. A normal heart rate is sixty.

Stress from training has two causes: either the duration of the training or the heart rate isn't adjusted to your own situation. With recovery training, you don't submit the body to any stress, so the accompanying local fatigue doesn't take place. You do, however, stimulate the body briefly to boost recovery speed. I recommend thirty-minute sessions with a ten-second speed-up every six minutes.

VACATION: A REST PERIOD?

A vacation allows you to leave everything behind for a while and unwind. Recovery training is ideal when traveling--you don't even need a gym. Walking, swimming, and cycling are perfect activities. If you decide not to exercise at all during your vacation, keep in mind that for every week of rest you need two weeks of exercise to get back up to your previous level. Once your body is rested, it's time to turn your workout up a notch.

TRAINING TOWARD A GOAL

Once you're rested--meaning your body experiences no stress--you can train toward a goal. Athletic goals can range from climbing a mountain to running a marathon. Health goals can be weight loss, a tighter body, diabetes prevention, physical rehabilitation after illness, or getting started again after a long period of no exercise.

Training toward a goal also consists of two phases.
The first phase is training for endurance. Endurance training takes place in the aerobic training zone, which means you get enough oxygen for your exertion. This is often referred to as talking speed, meaning that you can still talk during the exertion. Your aerobic system is maintained by the oxygen transport throughout your body, and it contributes to a healthy oxygen exchange between your organs. In other words, in this phase you train your cardiovascular system and oxygen transport. The longer you're able to train in the aerobic zone, the longer you're able to sustain an exertion. You're burning fat, and this reserve is practically inexhaustible. In addition, your heart rate goes down, which reduces the risk for heart disease. Everyone can benefit from this type of health training.

Having said that, endurance training isn't always what your body needs most. I see sprinters with busy jobs begin to slow down at some point. It could be the combination of long workdays and high pressure. They're physically fatigued, and a good short distance performance just isn't possible anymore. So they opt for marathon training. You get a pat on the back at the finish of a marathon regardless of how you got there. Unfortunately, simply changing your workout environment won't change the fact that your body doesn't perform optimally. Because of your endurance training your fatigue might not immediately register, and anyway, you can keep going on willpower alone, right? Or better yet, on adrenalin, though this supply is limited. That is how you set yourself up for a burnout.

To keep your body fit, it's important to provide a different burden during your training session than those it experiences during the day. It's perfectly fine to have an intense, short training session at the end of a long, monotonous, sleep-inducing day at the office. Conversely, it's better to opt for a calm recovery training after a stressful day. Longer endurance sessions are best left to the weekend or your days off, when you haven't had any work stress. You should determine your fatigue before a session—it helps you decide exactly what kind of training is ideal at that moment. This way you guard your health while at the same time increasing your vitality.

WHAT IS YOUR ANAEROBIC THRESHOLD

You could compare your anaerobic threshold to a car's fuel tank. When you raise your anaerobic threshold, you increase the size of your fuel tank. Your anaerobic threshold is the threshold where you start to gasp for breath and your body switches from burning fat to burning sugar. This means that at this level you're only be able to sustain the exertion for a short period of time. In this stage, you burn more carbohydrates (sugars) than fats, with lactic acid as the resulting waste. When you get enough oxygen, your body burns off the lactic acid. During anaerobic exercise, you don't get enough oxygen, and the lactic acid accumulates in your muscles, which leads to acidification. Result: You have a hard time keeping up the exercise because your speed, strength, and coordination decrease. The better trained you are, the longer it takes for you to reach this threshold and the longer you can sustain an exercise at a high intensity. Overweight or inactive people can sometimes reach this threshold when walking up stairs and other daily activities.

The second phase is training for enhanced fitness. In addition to endurance, you also train for agility, speed, strength, and muscle tone. They all help you sustain intense exertions for longer periods of time. You work on these with interval training in the anaerobic zone. During these anaerobic training sessions, you gasp for breath--you exercise with an oxygen deficit. This eventually raises your anaerobic threshold, so it takes longer to reach your limit. Interval training increases both your base speed and your heart and lungs' capacity. The idea is to switch rapidly between low and high intensity exertions, with the low intensity exertions being too short for complete recovery.

How do you know if you're ready for strength training? It depends on the condition of your central nervous system. The muscle system isn't all that smart. Sitting on a chair all day shortens your muscles, because your muscles simply carry out commands from the central nervous system. (More on this in Chapter 15.) When your central nervous system is fatigued, the commands it sends out travel slower, because the impulse transmission to the muscles is less efficient, and the result is a weaker muscle contraction. Strength training under these circumstances won't be efficient. It's best to start with recovery training. Stability exercises for a stronger core--your entire torso--are perfectly fine.

TRAINING IN BALANCE

Even when you train toward a goal, it's essential that you allow your body to recover. You have to find a balance between exertion and rest. Recovery training is appropriate after an exhausting day, but also after intense weight and cardio training. Walk or cycle for fifteen minutes directly after your session, and your stress and adrenalin levels will go down, which allows you to fall asleep easier later on.

A good training schedule that prepares you for a marathon or any other challenge takes rest into account. How long it takes you to recover from your training depends on your fitness level. It takes an average of fifteen hours after recovery training--after interval training it can be as much as 72 hours.

Classic training schedules work toward a concrete goal, for instance a 20K (12.5 miles). The road to such a goal is different for everyone, however. Your training schedule should consider your fitness level, but also your work and private life. Most training programs start with the question, "What is your goal?". Our program, on the other hand, starts with the question, "Are you rested?", which is the basis for effective performance training. And even at the starting blocks it's better to have a lower fitness level but a rested body than vice versa.

So a good training program is always based on the complete picture and always takes place according to your specific capacity. Your first exercise session might be a simple walk to stimulate your recovery, later on you might go jogging to develop your capacity for recovery, and in the end you may do interval training to enhance your fitness.

These are the different training zones:

- Recovery training (after a stressful day) = training as a means phase 1 – heart rate 60% of your maximum- 15 to 60 minutes.
- Endurance training = training as a means phase 2 – heart rate 70% of your maximum – 30 minutes and up.
- Endurance development = training toward a goal phase 1 – heart rate 80 to 85% of your maximum –45 to 90 minutes
- Endurance maintenance = training as a means phase 2 – heart rate 75 to 80% of your maximum – 1 to 4 hours
- Interval training = training toward a goal phase 2 – heart rate 95% of your maximum – 15 to 30 minutes, including rest periods
- Resistance training= training toward a goal phase 2 – heart rate 95 – 105% of your maximum – maximum 15 minutes

These training zones correlate with various energy systems discussed in Part Four. The heart rates are general, just to give you a basic guideline. You should always train in these zones based on your own maximum heart rate, which you should determine together with your personal trainer. And you should stay in the same heart rate zone your entire session. This gives your body the appropriate stimuli, and you exercise according to the appropriate energy system.

DETERMINING YOUR RESTING HEART RATE

A maximum stress test is not the best way to determine the heart rate zones for your fatigued body's recovery training, since it creates an extra stressor. Instead, work with a personal trainer who can determine your resting heart rate. You won't have to summon any extra motivation, and your fatigue, energy level and personal problems won't affect the measurements.

CHANGE IT UP

If you're like most people, you want to see the effects of training as soon as possible. You can accomplish this by giving your body training stimuli at unexpected times. Planning is important, but with the nuance that training is also about unexpected stress stimuli and new situations, because your body can get used to a certain exercise. Variation is key, especially when your time is limited.

A fifteen-minute walk once a day (morning, noon or night) has a much greater effect on your body than making the same rounds every Sunday evening.

Some of us are often still at work after midnight. In itself, this isn't abnormal or bad. You might have late shifts, or maybe you just like to work late because that's when you tend to get your best ideas and when you find solutions for ongoing problems. If you work late anyway, try scheduling the occasional low-intensity run with a measured heart rate before you hit the hay. You'll find that this has a big effect on your fitness, and the effect is even stronger with repeated nightly sessions. Most patients I see tell me they feel fitter for days afterward. Of course, they first determine their fatigue level to see if their body is ready for this.

CHAPTER 11:
WHICH SPORTS TYPE ARE YOU?

Your body carries the past with it. You should base your training on your fatigue, but also on your exercise history. When putting together a training plan, it's best to take into account the kind of sport or exercise you did when you were between twelve and twenty years old. You begin to develop your endurance around the age of twelve, and during the next eight years, while your body is still developing, you program yourself. You can program your body for sprints, for a technical sport, for endurance, or even for doing nothing at all. You can still teach yourself all these things when you are older--it just takes more effort.

NO SPORTS PAST

It's quite possible that your body never received any training stimuli before. In that case your inexperience makes it hard for you to recognize the signs of physical fatigue. After all, you have no frame of reference. If you experience your first physical discomfort while working out at the age of forty, for instance, it's important that you learn to check your fatigue level. You might not feel tired at all. Or, when lethargy makes your workout harder, you might blame your family dynamics, your financial situation, or business plans that aren't coming off the ground. Even though all these issues are definitely cause for concern, they do not cause your fatigue. When you have no sports past, your body never received training stimuli, and you never developed a strong physical capacity.

As mentioned earlier, at a later age—and compared to others your age— you may notice that you can't handle as much. You feel sluggish, tired, and occasionally short-fused. You want to change that, so you decide to join a gym, the local sports club, or get involved in a physical activity at work. In short, you hope exercise is your life saver, and that it will make you feel better. That's an excellent idea, but without the proper guidance you'll likely end up in a sports environment that doesn't take into account your fatigue, workload, or home situation.

The trainers—well-meaning though they are--tell you to immerse yourself in the sport with grit and determination. This is all new to you. Since the exertion accelerates circulation, adrenalin rushes through your body. You get more energy, but at the same time the first sessions feel like boot camp. Since you have no sports past, your body's recovery capacity is low and you don't feel at your best in the beginning. You manage to keep it up for a while, but after six weeks the fatigue has begun to accumulate. You no longer recover and you feel like quitting. You're fighting yourself—you have muscle aches, trouble sleeping, you consume more sugar, etc.

At this point the big question is: do you really want to try to sustain this, and let yourself be swept along by the goals of the group? Is sport really the right goal for you? Or would it be better to exercise as a means to improve your health, without having to go to the limit? In my experience sport as a means to improve your health is usually best, starting with recovery training. Be sure to get proper guidance, because you don't have the experience to know what to expect from an exercise session. Talk with your trainer about your goals and your fatigue. Learn to recognize what's happening in your body, and use a heart rate monitor to measure the intensity of your workout. To begin with, a ten to fifteen-minute recovery training four times a week, at different times of day, is ideal. Choose something like walking or swimming. Once you get going, and if your body allows, you can switch to training toward a goal.

A SPRINTING PAST

If you were a sprinter in your youth, you're used to living in high gear. You're conditioned to develop the largest possible capacity in a very short time. This required high adrenalin levels and you enjoyed the accompanying kick. At a later age, you tend to look for sports that give you a similar high.

When you prepare for a training session, your body goes into elevated performance mode even before the actual physical activity. During your session, you subject yourself to a short but powerful stress response. You put the pedal to the metal, you give it your all, hoping for a good performance time. For fuel, you use creatine phosphate--which is as quickly consumed as it is delivered. Your brakes, on the other hand, aren't trained at all well. You don't always realize when you're stressed or when your adrenalin level is high.

This combination can lead to fatigue, so the first step to good health is recovery training and developing your recovery time. Do mild endurance training, but tailored to your sprinter past, not according to the rules of training science. Don't do long sessions--twenty to thirty minutes is enough. After all, aerobic exertion has its effect on the body of an ex-sprinter much sooner than on someone with a past in endurance or game sports.

A PAST IN BALL GAMES

If you're a ball player (football, soccer, basketball, baseball, etc.) you're conditioned to carry out a wide variety of movements--from short sprints to running or even walking--and you're capable of sustaining an intense exertion for up to ninety minutes. Yet, training that requires sustaining the same pace for a long time bores you. You prefer activities with regular changes in tempo, and you're always looking for different stimuli. Since you experience adrenalin as a positive drug, you tend to overdo your training. Your sessions are usually long, which can lead to hormonal fatigue. When developing your recovery speed, you should insert ten to fifteen-second spurts every ten minutes. They stimulate your system without tiring you out.

A PAST IN ENDURANCE SPORTS

In Belgium, the best-known endurance sport you can get involved in at a relatively young age is cycling. Cycling sessions usually occur below your maximum performance level, so you can keep them up longer. You also strongly stimulate your recovery--your body's brakes. In other words, you're conditioned to recover as quickly as possible when you're running on empty, so you probably don't experience the damaging impact of acute stress later in life. Endurance should obviously be the basis for your training program.

However, if you have too many long endurance sessions, you become over-trained. Your main risk is hormonal fatigue, which brings morning lethargy and apathy with it. Because you're used to training for long periods at the same pace, getting your body out of its regular pattern makes you stronger. That means: many stimuli and regular changes in tempo.

CHAPTER 12:
TAILORED TRAINING PLAN

TRAINING WHEN YOU'RE PHYSICALLY FATIGUED

When you're physically fatigued, training toward a specific goal may still be possible in the short run, but once you're done you feel tired and sluggish, so it's hard to stay motivated.

Start off with recovery training. Train three to four times a week for ten to thirty minutes at a low intensity, keeping your heart rate under your anaerobic level (at talking speed). Start with ten minutes and add two minutes every week. This recovery usually takes six to eight weeks.

Choose individual sports like swimming, walking or cycling. Don't bring music because the lively beat can tempt you to increase your pace, which would get you back into adrenalin mode.

Ask yourself why you exercise. Do you do it because of a physical or a social need? Question your urge to work out, and allow yourself to listen to the signals your fatigued body gives you.

Don't switch to more intense training, or a game sport until you feel energetic again during the workday. Only a well-rested body can deal with intense training stimuli. When you've had a hard day at work, opt for recovery training in the evening. In fact, don't give your body intense training stimuli after being awake for fourteen hours, whether you've had a hard day or not. If you train at a leisurely pace, you don't add to the burden of your fatigued body, and you should fall asleep easily.

TRAINING WHEN YOU'RE HORMONALLY FATIGUED

When you're hormonally fatigued, your endocrine function is disrupted, so it takes you longer to recover from training. Your adrenal gland, may be affected by medication, diet, and intense training programs.

To begin with, focus on improving your recovery speed. Running, cycling or swimming three to four times a week is ideal. Focus on short sessions— thirty minutes, tops. Varying your speed helps boost recovery—insert ten-second speed increases every five minutes. Your heart rate goes up during the acceleration. Measure how long it takes you to be back at your base value. Then continue at your base tempo.

Morning training activates your body. Don't do it every day, though, because between 7:00 and 9:00 am your adrenal gland is still recovering. Stimulate your neurological system every now and then. Sprint up the stairs for two to three minutes, for instance. This increases your alertness, it makes your blood flow, and it activates your energy system.

Do mild strength training to maintain your core. Train your belly and back muscles in short series of eight to ten repetitions. You should wait with doing more advanced strength training until you're fully recovered—if not, you'll exhaust your adrenal gland even more.

TIP
Evaluate regularly and adjust your action plan as needed.
Depending on your main issues, your symptoms, or your state of recovery, advice for hormonal fatigue could eventually need to change to advice for physical fatigue. What you do today might not work six months from now. The advice is temporary and functions as a life saver, so you don't continue to destroy your body. They are meant to get you started on a path that helps you be healthy for as long as possible.

TRAINING WHEN YOU'RE MENTALLY FATIGUED

When you're mentally fatigued, you may lack the motivation to exercise intensely for long periods of time. Build it up gradually, skip the recovery training, and focus on improving your recovery speed. Walking, cycling and swimming are ideal.

Don't set the bar too high. Don't go for any ambitious, intense training programs. (But do follow clear guidelines. If you only train based on how you feel, you won't improve much.) Don't do any strength, technique or coordination training--the effects are minimal.

Your tendency to procrastinate requires a low exercise threshold. Don't say things like "I have to exercise". Try to focus on relaxation. If possible, train in a quiet environment, like a forest, where you can enjoy the fresh air. Plan relatively short sessions, lasting between 30 and 45 minutes, and stay below the anaerobic threshold. Is even thirty minutes too long for you? Don't worry--fifteen minutes still makes a difference. The important thing is that you're taking the first step to making exercise a habit. In the end all these little bits do make a difference. Reward yourself for training and for sticking to it.

TRAINING WHEN YOU'RE METABOLICALLY FATIGUED

When you're metabolically fatigued, you have been reaching deep into your reserves during your prolonged stress without realizing it, and now your tank is empty.

Aim for complete recovery of your energy systems. Start with aerobic training at talking speed. It encourages the delivery of oxygen to your organs. Include short accelerations that stimulate your anaerobic energy system. This way your muscles won't acidify as quickly.

Limit the length of your sessions and keep your heart rate low. Alternate between training stimuli and adequate recovery. You don't have the energy for strength training or explosive stress stimuli. Wait with these until your energy systems have recovered.

Because your metabolic fatigue is almost always a combination of various forms of physical and hormonal fatigue, and since it occurs after a period of prolonged stress, personalized advice is an absolute must.

LET'S RECAP

1. When you're fatigued and you want to start exercising, **be aware of your fatigue**. When you give an already fatigued body even more stressors, in the long run, you will inevitably suffer from exhaustion, burnout, depression, etc.

2. **Moving is a basic need**. It provides much-needed relaxation, and it keeps your muscles and joints supple. Specialists recommend getting up and stretching your legs every thirty minutes, and actually moving at least thirty minutes per day.

3. When you start **to exercise**, it's important to get a personal trainer to help you put together a program tailored to your fatigue and level of fitness at the start, and that includes rest and recovery. A good personal trainer is expensive, but so is the price you pay if your body slowly deteriorates.

4. **Training** is carried out according to the laws of training science and exertion physiology. With an individual program tailored to your needs, your training is based on certain heart rate zones, aimed at reaching specific goals.

5. **Tiring out the body** through interval training or any other type of exercise is only recommended for a rested body. When you're not fully recovered from previous stressors and you have no rest in your private and/or work life, you must do recovery training first.

6. **Recovery training** consists of two phases. The first phase results in a rested body, the second phase develops your body's ability to recover.

7. Once you're rested--meaning your body experiences no stress--you can **train toward a goal**. The first phase is training for endurance; the second phase is training for enhanced fitness.

8. **Your body carries the past with it**. You should base your training on your fatigue, but also on your exercise history. The kind of sport or exercise you did when you were between twelve and twenty years old determines how your body is programmed.

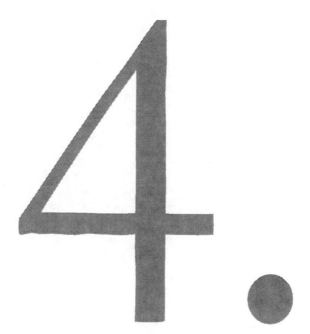

UNDERSTANDING YOUR BODY

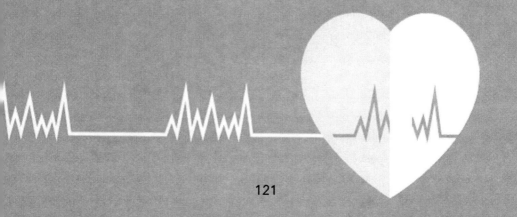

This section explains the critical body processes. When you have a good understanding of your body, you can make the right decisions when you perceive fatigue signals. First, we'll look at what really happens in your body when you're tired. Then we'll discuss where you get your energy from, and we'll take a closer look at neuro-transmitters—the brain's messengers. Finally, we'll look at how your body keeps itself balanced: we'll explore the key elements of your biochemistry and immunity.

CHAPTER 13:
THE PHYSICAL PROCESSES
BEHIND FATIGUE

In Part One we described the triggers and symptoms of the four types of fatigue. In the following we take it a step further by delving into the physical processes.

UNDERSTANDING PHYSICAL FATIGUE

Physical fatigue occurs when there's a constant imbalance between the components of your autonomic nervous system. The autonomic nervous system monitors all the functions you don't have to think about. It works independently and instinctively. Via an electric circuit, it automatically regulates the critical physical activities for your survival: your heartbeat, respiration, digestion, and metabolic rate.

This in contrast to your central nervous system, which allows you to carry out actions and commands--moving, speaking, memory, and decision-making. Professor Boudewijn Van Houdenhove, psychiatrist and Professor Medical and Health Psychology at the Catholic University in Leuven, Belgium, describes the three components of the autonomic nervous system as follows:

The sympathetic nervous system is responsible for our fight-or-flight response. Both physical stressors (like exertions, temperature changes, pain, and noise) and emotional stressors (like pressure and startling events) can evoke this response. Your adrenal glands secrete adrenalin and noradrenalin, two stress hormones that enable your vital organs--heart, lungs, muscles, etc.--to jump into action lightning fast. Your muscles are activated, your heart rate and breathing quicken, your pupils widen, and your skin pales because the blood is going to your heart, muscles, and brain. Your digestion is on the backburner because that's hardly relevant in a fight-or-flight situation. Your blood glucose level, on the other hand, is high, so your focus is great. You also sweat, even at low temperatures, and time seems to move more slowly. In short: you're ready for action.

The visceral-afferent system lets you feel these physical changes through heart palpitations, nausea, etc. The nerve fibers of this system receive messages which they relay to the central nervous system. It's a way for your central nervous system to make sure you've got the message: it's flight-or-fight time.

The parasympathetic system counters your sympathetic system. It allows your vital organs to calm down once the threat is gone. Your heart rate and blood pressure drop, your muscles and organs get plenty of blood and oxygen, and your digestion goes back to work. Your body is no longer on hair-trigger alert and you can carry on as usual.

You could compare your sympathetic system to the gas pedal and your parasympathetic system with the brake pedal. It's exactly this brake pedal that's key to health in general, and recovery in particular. When resting, you usually have your foot on the brake pedal. When you experience physical or emotional stress, you let up on the brakes a little. This happens, for instance, after a difficult meeting or a one-hour workout, but it can also happen while walking the dog or simply getting out of bed. The last two examples may not seem stressful by themselves, but every impulse makes you ease off the brakes a little. This is how your sympathetic system can adapt to the changing circumstances and support your activities without having to call on the extreme fight-or-flight response. Your parasympathetic brake mechanism keeps an eye out so you stay in balance.

Here's another analogy. Let's say you have a bucket with water. The sympathetic system adds water to the bucket—small amounts at a time, but they could add up and cause the bucket to overflow eventually. Fortunately, the parasympathetic system is like a scoop that regularly takes a scoop of water out of the bucket, so it doesn't overflow. When the systems aren't in balance, the odds are bigger that the bucket overflows: stress gets a hold of you.

When this happens, your sympathetic system takes over and your fight-or-flight responses follow each other in quick succession. You feel constantly rushed and you go into overdrive. In this situation, even the slightest stimulus can cause you to overreact. For instance, when you want to make a quick trip to the grocery store after a hard day at work, and you get stuck in bumper to bumper traffic. Then even a long line at the checkout counter can cause you a lot of stress.

Your metaphorical gas and brake pedals work for both physical and emotional stress. Overuse of either leads to an imbalance. Like hypersensitive people, you experience a physical overreaction to stress. Your hypothalamus—the brain section that watches over your internal balance—becomes confused and is no longer able to process your internal information correctly.

This is why, you become oversensitive to stimuli. Even the slightest light, noise or an inappropriate remark bother you. You might also experience neck pain, headache, chest pain, dizziness, and heart palpitations, as well as a dry mouth and loss of appetite. Sweating, hyperventilation, and trouble sleeping are also included in this complaint package. These discomforts occur acutely. When detected on time, adequate sleep, relaxation, and a healthy diet can usually get you back to normal soon. But if the situation continues and you don't get enough rest, your body steps in and decides to slam on the brakes. Physically you feel sluggish and mentally you feel tired and dazed all day. If you feel like this often, your physical discomfort can lead to mental discomfort as well. After all, you start worrying about your health.

UNDERSTANDING HORMONAL FATIGUE

The word 'hormone' is Greek for 'driving force', and that is exactly what hormones are for your body. They are involved in your mental health, cell production, and metabolism, among many other things. Hormonal fatigue occurs after a prolonged period of physical or emotional stress.

In Chapter 2, we looked at the stress response known as the fight-or-flight response. The hypothalamus--the brain section that manages your autonomic nervous system and your endocrine system--manages this stress response. It keeps watch. It springs into action when you respond to stress and it puts a stop to it all once the danger has subsided.

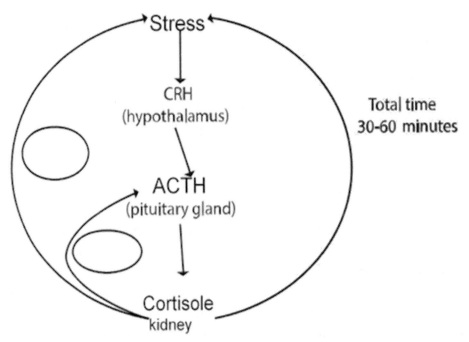

IMAGE 6 The hypothalamic pituitary axis

When there's an unexpected event or threat, your body responds quickly and explosively. The hypothalamus tells your adrenal glands to secrete adrenalin. It used to happen when confronted with a charging lion on the savanna, and now it happens when you're driving and you suddenly have to slam on the brakes, or when a co-worker attacks you personally and out of the blue. Symptoms of your response in these situations are rapid breathing, higher energy level, and excessive sweating.

Under normal circumstances your stress system can turn itself off again. For instance, when you've narrowly avoided a car accident, it's normal to be catching your breath for some time afterward, and to feel your heart pound. Fifteen minutes later you're usually back to normal. After all, your stress response ends as soon as the threat goes away. It's exactly this shifting down, this recovery, that suffers under prolonged stress.

A charging lion is an acute but temporary threat. The problem is that our present-day challenges last longer, they pile up, and flight is not an option. They're related to job pressure, rush hour traffic, unpaid bills, human conflicts, insecurities, illness, etc. When a coworker verbally attacks you during a meeting, you feel ready to burst, but you have no way out because a meeting room isn't the savannah. However, your stress system can't tell the difference between one undesired stressor (a charging lion), and another—regardless of the stressor, it responds in the same way. And so you end up using the fight-or-flight response--which was meant for short, acute threat situations--almost constantly in your daily life. When this happens, you suffer from chronic stress.

When you drive your car and you constantly rev up, you're driving inefficiently. You overburden the car, and if you don't slow down, the engine ends up overheating. Similarly, your body can't handle being constantly in fight-or-flight mode. Perhaps you ignore the problem, or you overestimate yourself, or perhaps you're just not sufficiently aware of your body's signals. Either way, your problems seem never-ending and you can't find a way out. You rarely have the opportunity, to go through the entire stress cycle. This includes:

- Stressor
- Decision to fight or flee
- Action
- Rest

YOUR ENDOCRINE SYSTEM

Hormones are chemical substances that influence slow processes, like your metabolism, growth and behavior. Via the bloodstream they reach and then enter the target cells or organs, to convey their message. The endocrine system contains several hormone-producing organs:

- Hypothalamus and pituitary gland (detection system)
- Thyroid and parathyroid gland (metabolism)
- Adrenal gland (stress hormones)
- Pancreas (insulin)
- Reproductive glands (reproductive hormones like testosterone and estrogen)

Hormones are chemicals that influence the slow processes, like your metabolism, growth, and behavior. They reach the target cells or organs via the blood stream, to deliver their messages.

The hypothalamus detects this ongoing stress, and it knows that additional energy is needed. It tells your pituitary gland to tell your adrenal gland to get to work. The hypothalamus releases hormones into the blood stream that tell the pituitary gland to relay information to the adrenal gland. When the pituitary gland gets the message, it also releases hormones into the blood stream. When the adrenal gland gets the message, it starts to produce the stress hormone cortisol.

Cortisol gives you a constant energy supply, and it aids the adrenalin in your blood. In the first stage of cortisol secretion, your metabolic rate and blood glucose levels rise, and you might lose weight. Your immune function also improves at first--wounds and infections heal fast. But after a while your digestion, your immunity and your libido slow down as the cortisol reserves your energy for more immediate threats.

Because so much adrenalin and cortisol is running through your blood, your recovery mechanism no longer works the way it should. Your endocrine system--the hormone-regulating system--becomes less sensitive. In other words, you get used to the many stressors coming at you, so your body no longer puts the brakes on your stress response. You're ready to flee or fight all the time and your stress response only stops after extreme stressors. Only when your body finally slams on the brakes and gives up, does your system detect this extreme stress, and you feel fatigued. By that time, it's usually too late. You've been running on empty too long to recover any time soon.

If this is the case, you suffer from hormonal fatigue, and it can have serious consequences. Your constantly elevated blood glucose can lead to type 2 diabetes, your high blood pressure can lead to cardiovascular problems, metabolism problems can lead to extreme weight loss or gain, and overstimulation of the neurological system in combination with muscle tension can lead to disc hernia.

UNDERSTANDING MENTAL FATIGUE

To understand how mental fatigue works, we must take a peek inside the brain. After all, your brain and your emotions have tremendous influence on your hormonal and other body functions and vice versa. The human brain consists of two large, separate structures which barely impact each other--the limbic system (our emotional brain) and the neocortex (our rational brain).

The limbic system is the primitive brain. It evolved with the arrival of birds and mammals. Unlike earlier animal types like fish and reptiles, whose young are on their own once they hatch, young birds and most mammals are completely helpless for quite a while after birth. Their parents provide food and care, and they only become independent, later on. So, the limbic system contains a group of brain structures that together are responsible for emotions, moods, motivation, memory, pleasure, and sexual behavior, all attributes that are necessary for basic survival.

MILLIONS OF YEARS-THREE BRAINS

To understand why our emotions are so important and why we often act emotionally and even instinctively—against our better judgment—we refer you to American neurologist Paul MacLean's theory of the triune brain. The idea is that our brain consists of three sections which each developed in different stages of evolution.

The reptile brain came first in evolution, about 500 million years ago. It monitors your critical body functions as well as your survival instinct, including aggression, dominance, eating, drinking, breathing, procreation and sleep. This area of your brain is located near your brain stem and it responds lightning fast.

The limbic system developed later. It increases our survival chances through emotions like fear and love, as well as recall, learning processes and memory.

The neocortex arose some 100, 000 years ago. Although your reason represents tons of brain power, our instincts and emotions still dominate in tricky situations. These systems are more deeply embedded in our responses.

Of all mammals, humans are the most helpless at birth and for the longest time afterward. Parents need to have a long, emotional bond with their children, in order to increase their survival chances. This is a subconscious thing, separate from thinking. You automatically bond with others and send the necessary messages because your limbic brain runs your emotions. This emotional communication is essential. A baby asks for attention from its parents by crying, and the parents respond, thus increasing its chances of survival. Reptiles and fish don't have the limbic brain, which explains why you're capable of immediately having an emotional connection with a cat or a dog, but not so much with a fish or a snake.

These are your limbic brain's main structures and their functions:

- The amygdala is responsible for summoning and processing several emotions, like aggression and fear.
- The hippocampus is related to recall.
- The hypothalamus runs your endocrine system. It monitors your internal balance and plays a key role in regulating the autonomic nervous system. It prepares you for action and it takes care of recovery. It also regulates your biological clock and your energy system via messages of hunger, thirst or satisfaction. So, it covers all your basic needs.
- The pituitary gland is a protrusion of the hypothalamus.

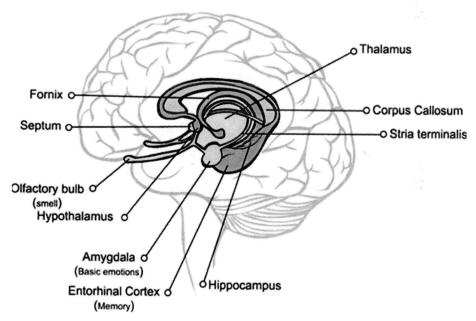

IMAGE 7 The limbic system

The neocortex showed up millions of years after the limbic system. It's the newest component of our brain. Although all mammals have a neocortex, the human neocortex is the most evolved. The prefrontal cortex is located behind your forehead, above your eyes. This area of the brain is a whiz at processing information. It's your rational brain and it gives you all your reasoning skills: language, reason, memory, focus and concentration, planning, decision making, etc.

Since your emotional and rational brains developed at vastly different times in evolution, they work completely differently. Your limbic system has a rougher structure than the neocortex. It processes information at a much more primitive level. That's not a problem, because the information processing in your limbic system is focused on your survival, so it happens fast and directly. This system doesn't analyze--it summons up immediate survival responses. If you had to first analyze all the aspects of a dangerous situation, chances are your deliberated response to the situation would come way too late. For instance, think of the startle response when an object suddenly comes flying at you. Whether it's a sponge or a brick, you duck without thinking.

EMOTIONS IN YOUR BODY AND BRAIN

Although your emotional and rational brains work independently from each other, they do influence each other. Portuguese neurologist Antonio Damasio discovered that sadness causes a decrease in activity in your prefrontal cortex, happiness causes an increase. So good vibes are not a myth. Activities in the prefrontal cortex are a strong indicator for ideas and lively thoughts. When you're on high alert, full of ideas, your prefrontal lobes work at full tilt. But Damasio also goes a step further. He believes your visceral-afferent system in your autonomic nervous system is the basis for your emotional life. Without goosebumps, increased heart rate, trembling lips, churning stomach, little would be left of your emotions (except fear?)

Your emotional and rational brains work independently of each other. At best, they are able to keep each other in check. You recall from Chapter 3 that mental fatigue can cause you to either suppress your emotions or give them free rein in response to overstimulation. This disrupts your endocrine system. It can also lead to physical fatigue symptoms.

YOUR GUT – YOUR SECOND BRAIN

The enteric nervous system is a bundle of nerve cells. It runs from the esophagus to the anus. The nerves in the pancreas, the gallbladder and the bile ducts are also controlled by this system. We are talking about more than ten million nerve cells—more than the number of nerve cells in your spinal cord. This is why, it's also known as the *little brain*. It exchanges information with the central nervous system via the autonomic nervous system. This explains why you feel butterflies in your belly when you're in love and it makes you lose your appetite.

UNDERSTANDING METABOLIC FATIGUE

Your metabolism is the process of transforming nutrients into energy. Metabolic fatigue occurs when the process is disrupted due to prolonged stress, with less energy as a result. It's a specific type of fatigue, and though it usually occurs in combination with other forms of fatigue, you mustn't underestimate its importance. The stress hormones do supply the necessary energy, so it seems like you can still handle everything. This is how your tank gradually empties. You begin to feel sluggish during heavy physical activity. If you keep going on willpower in this situation, you only make things worse. Complete recovery from metabolic fatigue is extremely slow.

During a period of prolonged stress, you use up more nutrients. Your body is focused on consuming and less on regenerating. You don't sleep enough because the stress response keeps you awake, and the digestive organs receive less blood than your muscles, heart, and lungs, because the latter get priority during a fight-or-flight event. As a result, your body only partially absorbs the necessary nutrients, even if you eat enough healthy food. That may not be the case, though, because your body doesn't give off hunger signals during times of stress.

Your metabolism is in a downward spiral: you consume *more* nutrients, but you don't *absorb* enough, so your tank slowly empties out. Life spent with the pedal to the metal jeopardizes your energy reserves.

Stress responses also have an impact on body's acidity. Your stomach acid is affected, so certain nutrients enter your intestines only half digested, and bad bacteria end up in your intestines, which adds to your stress. Prolonged fatigue also disrupts the acid levels elsewhere in your body. The result is a lot of waste, acid, and toxic substances, which makes the energy exchange between your cells more difficult.

YOUR THYROID - EXTRA HELP?

Apart from causing the adrenalin shots in your autonomic nervous system and the extra cortisol production in your adrenal gland, your thyroid is an extra link in the chain reaction of persistent fatigue. This butterfly-shaped gland that's barely 1.5 in tall and 2.3 in wide is located at the front of your neck and it regulates your energy level at rest. It does this by checking your metabolic rate. When your adrenal gland is on the verge of exhaustion, your thyroid tries to fix things by producing more thyroid hormone in order to keep the right energy level via metabolism. This causes excessive sweating, heart palpitations, and feeling anxious and unstable. Your thyroid gives up rather soon, so you don't quite have the right amount of thyroid hormone. Your base energy level drops, which leaves you fatigued, especially when rising in the morning. You have a hard time getting started, your muscles and joints feel stiff, and you can't think clearly. These are just a random few of the many symptoms.

When your energy cache is depleted, your body switches to an emergency measure, gluconeogenesis. This process occurs mostly in the liver. Here non-carbohydrates such as proteins and lactic acid are converted into glucose. But unlike the normal absorption of carbohydrates, this process takes energy. So, periods of stress and intense workouts, combined with an untailored diet, can eventually lead to metabolic fatigue.

CHAPTER 14:
YOUR ENERGY CONSUMPTION

As you now know, it's all about the energy. As the gas in your tank is not unlimited, so do your body's energy stores have limits. Timely refueling is key. Your car needs gas--your body needs food. Your total energy usage is a combination of three factors: your resting metabolic rate, exercise, and digestion.

Your resting metabolic rate is your energy usage while at rest. It accounts for 60 to 70% of your energy usage. You use energy even when you're resting, to let all the bodily functions run smoothly. Since muscles use more energy than fat, and men have more muscle mass, men on average use 5 to 10% more energy at rest than women. An underactive thyroid decreases your resting metabolic rate, as does aging. For every ten years you age, you lose 2 to 3% of your muscle mass.

Thermogenesis is the amount of warmth energy your body emits during food absorption and digestion. This accounts for approximately 10% of your total energy usage and it's determined by what you eat. The extra energy that your body needs to keep warm also increases your thermogenesis, as do medicines and nutrients like caffeine.

Exercise: All forms of exercise also count, of course, so that includes household activities and office work. On average exercise accounts for 10 to 30% of your total energy usage. If you train intensely, this component increases. A Tour de France cyclist can even use 70% of his energy this way. Athletes move more, so their many muscles burn more calories during physical exertion. Heavier people also burn more when they move, since they carry more weight along. But even when you're tired, you need more energy for the same physical exertion, for instance walking stairs, much like a car drives at a higher rpm if you never let up on the accelerator.

Another way your body uses energy related to exercise is Excess Post Oxygen Consumption (EPOC). When you exercise for a short period of time at high intensity and in a high heart rate range, your body continues to take in oxygen after the workout, using the extra energy to recover and stabilize. Your metabolic rate stays high for up to 72 hours after your workout. The new fitness rage—short intense 20-minute workouts, or HIITT workouts (High Intensity Interval Training) is based on this process.

CALORIES

A calorie denotes the energy value of a nutrient. It's how you can measure how many calories you take in daily. On average, women require 2,000 calories a day, men need 2,500 calories. Of course, everything depends on how much energy you burn per day. Your body stores the excess as fat and doesn't use it until you have a calorie debit. So, in general, the more calories you consume, the more weight you can gain.

But not all calories are equal. Calories only tell us about the energy value, nothing about the nutritional value. One hundred ml whiskey, for instance, has 243 calories and 100 g chips even has 493 calories, without giving you any of the necessary nutrients, minerals or vitamins. That's why the calories in alcohol, soda, chips, etc. are called empty calories. Fats and alcohol also contain more calories per gram than proteins and carbohydrates: carbohydrates and proteins provide 4 calories/g, alcohol 7 calories/g and fat 9 calories/g. To give you an idea: one 100 g beef has 280 calories—about half the calories of 100 g chips--but it's high in protein.

A calorie also tells us nothing about portions or the level of satisfaction you feel after eating. You can still handle a full meal after a glass of whiskey or a handful of chips, while you feel more satisfied after eating a portion of meat.

The timing of your calorie intake is also essential. Calories consumed in the morning are a better deal than those consumed in the evening, since you can burn them during your daily activities.

And finally, it's important to know that your digestion and your ability to actually absorb nutrients also play a role. Our digestion isn't one hundred percent efficient. When you're in balance, you get about 97, 95 and 92% energy respectively from carbohydrates, fats and protein. But fiber and protein reduce digestive efficiency, so you absorb less energy from your food. If you're fatigued or stressed, you also get less energy from food, because the stress response puts your digestion on the back burner. Inefficient digestion can lead to metabolic fatigue, which in turn also prevents you from getting enough energy from food, despite your healthy diet.

THE THREE ENERGY SYSTEMS

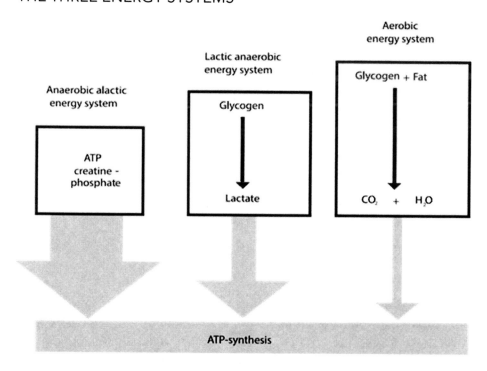

The three energy systems
IMAGE 8 The three energy systems

Food gives you energy for exercise and your bodily functions. You get this energy from carbohydrates (sugars) and fats. Your body can't immediately use this energy--first it has to change the chemical energy from your food into bio-energy, or ATP (adenosine triphosphate). You don't keep all the ATP immediately available because it's a relatively heavy molecule. Just keeping it at the ready all the time would cost your body way too much energy. That's why ATP in turn gets converted into different forms, which are changed back into ATP only when needed.

The three different forms of converted ATP are stored in various parts of your body. Depending on the intensity of exertion, your body turns on one of three different energy systems.

ATP-PC System

For very short and powerful energy bursts, your body turns on the system that uses the energy that's immediately available: pure ATP, stored in your muscles. ATP isn't an efficient fuel and you don't get much more than ten seconds' worth, so if more is needed after ten seconds, this system uses energy that's stored as phosphocreatine (PC for short). It converts the phosphocreatine back to ATP without using oxygen and without producing lactic acid. Phosphocreatine gives you another ten to twenty seconds--good for a sprint, for instance. So the ATP-PC system is quite an energy bomb. And although it's only available for some thirty seconds, you quickly refill your store during a rest interval. After no more than 20 to 25 seconds rest, your tank is already half full again. The ATP-PC system is also referred to as the anaerobic alactic energy system, because it doesn't use oxygen and it doesn't produce lactic acid.

Anaerobic system

The anaerobic system provides you with slightly less intense, slightly longer bursts of energy that can last up to about two minutes. This system is good for a sprint, for instance. The anaerobic system converts glycogen (glucose stored in your liver and muscles) back to ATP. It's also referred to as the anaerobic lactic system, because it doesn't use oxygen to convert the glycogen, but it does produce lactic acid. Result: your muscles acidify and after a while they have a hard time contracting. That is your body's way of telling you that you should take it a little easier. The lactic acid is your personal brake pedal, as it were.

Aerobic system

This system consists of two stages.

In the first stage—**aerobic glycolysis**--the system uses oxygen to convert glycogen back to ATP. Your body can keep up a lower-intensity exertion for longer periods of time using this system, because it converts the glycogen to ATP *while you exercise*. The aerobic system gets you 45 to 90 minutes--even longer if you have an energy drink. It's ideal for spinning class or game sports like soccer or tennis.

The more you exercise, the bigger the store of glycogen becomes, so the later the switch from aerobic to anaerobic energy burning occurs (when you start to huff and puff). For instance, an athlete can keep using the aerobic system for an entire marathon, while someone with less training can get out of breath at a much lower intensity, huffing and puffing after running one kilometer. In that case, when your body realizes that the activity is more intense, it switches up to the anaerobic energy systems.

The second stage is the **oxidative stage**, in which the system uses oxygen to convert fat back to ATP. Your fat reserves are almost endless, so this stage allows you to sustain a long, continuous activity. Since it's aerobic, it is used in continuous activity that is *low-intensity*, when you breathe regularly and you can still talk. A typical activity for burning fat is walking. When you're in bad shape, or you increase the intensity of your exertion for some other reason, your body shifts up to the anaerobic systems, and you suppress your fat-burning.

We have described the three energy systems separately for clarity's sake. In reality, they work together, with each system being more or less active. They depend on one another, because the chemicals produced by ATP burning in one system get used in another system to create ATP anew.

CHAPTER 15: NEUROTRANSMITTERS

For a holistic approach, we can't forget neurotransmitters. Neurotransmitters are chemicals that allow your brain to send messages from one nerve cell to the next. They provide the chemistry, and therefore the electrical activity or impulse transmission in your brain. So, it's obvious that neurotransmitters can also cause your fatigue, apathy, and even depression—in other words, your body chemistry can determine your feelings.

WHAT ARE NEUROTRANSMITTERS?

Neurons—nerve cells--are located throughout your body. The neurons in your brain are involved in conveying information to your senses and in driving the muscles. Although neurons are great in receiving, processing, and sending on information, they can't directly communicate with one another. That's where neurotransmitters come in.

Like testosterone, estrogen, and cortisol, some neurotransmitters are hormones. The big difference between neurotransmitters and other hormones is that hormones work in the entire body, while neurotransmitters usually don't. They emit their messages via tiny channels or structures, often referred to as neural pathways. That way they're sure they don't circulate over unnecessarily long distances, which would affect the speed of the message delivery.

When the neurotransmitter encounters the neuron's specific receptor, or antenna, an electrical signal—the message--is created. This happens at the synapse. The neurotransmitter sends the message off, further along your nervous system, through the neural pathways. When the neurotransmitter has done its job, one of two things happens: either it's reabsorbed by its neuron and thus stays in circulation, or it's broken down by an enzyme.

The messages neurotransmitters send regulate, among other things, your mood, appetite, sleep, and pain response. So, it's no surprise that the state of your neurotransmitters can affect your mental and your physical health.

These are the conditions for optimal neurotransmission:
- Sufficient oxygen (and therefore blood) to the brain
- A stable blood glucose level
- Sufficient omega-3 fatty acids in your brain
- Enough vitamins and minerals

These are factors that can disrupt neurotransmission:
- Hormonal imbalance and a cortisol excess
- An underactive thyroid
- Certain molds and intestinal parasites can also cause disruptions from a distance, among others certain brain functions

THE CHEMISTRY BEHIND YOUR PLEASURE, BREAK AND GAS PEDAL

Although your body has various neurotransmitters, we will limit our discussion to serotonin, dopamine, and GABA. Together they are responsible for your sleep, energy, and rest, respectively—they are the basic elements of your body's gas and brake pedals. So are adrenalin and noradrenalin neurotransmitters, but we discussed those in the previous chapter.

Serotonin

Although 80% of your serotonin, is located in the intestines and is linked to intestinal problems, serotonin also has a major effect on various brain functions.
- It affects your mood, so it contributes to your happiness. For instance, serotonin makes you feel calm and slightly euphoric. A serotonin deficiency can cause opposite feelings like depression, fear, restlessness, irritability, mood swings, and a lower pain threshold.

- It also affects your sex, so a deficiency causes a reduced libido.
- It affects your eating habits, so a deficiency causes a craving for sweets.
- It regulates your sleep. It plays a role in the production of the antioxidant hormone melatonin. Melatonin is involved in your sleep functions and it's produced by the pineal gland in your brain. Melatonin determines your biological clock, so it should come as no surprise that it's sensitive to light. Both sunlight and artificial light boost the production of serotonin, while darkness spurs the conversion of serotonin into melatonin. A serotonin deficiency can lead to sleeplessness.
- It also affects many other neurotransmitters, including noradrenalin, dopamine, and endorphin. For instance, serotonin is responsible for an increased production of endorphins, your natural feel-good drug.

How do you increase the levels? Serotonin levels, are stimulated by the amino acid tryptophan. (More on amino acids and proteins in Chapter 5.) Tryptophan produces serotonin via vitamins B and C. It can also be found in avocados and bananas. It's best to minimize your intake of refined sugars. The extra dose of the hormone insulin, which regulates your blood glucose levels, can lead to hormonal imbalance. As a result, your body is less efficient in producing serotonin. Stress--and especially cortisol--is the culprit, because it stops tryptophan from stimulating more serotonin. Sunlight and human skin contact also have a positive effect on serotonin. When you have trouble falling asleep, an evening walk is ideal.

WHICH STRATEGY DO YOU USE?

The brake and gas pedals are the key elements of your autonomic nervous system. American researcher Stephan Porges adds a third element with his Polyvagal Theory: the social system. According to this theory you check the following strategy list when a threat occurs:

• Your social system: communication, love, empathy, team work, group action, and psychology are appropriate strategies nowadays to deal with threats.
• Your sympathetic nervous system (gas pedal): if the first strategy doesn't work, you switch to the second. You fall back on the old fight-or-flight response.

Your parasympathetic nervous system (brake pedal): hitting the brakes is a strategy as well. You play dead and hope the threat goes away. If this third strategy doesn't work either, you are in mortal danger

Of course, a fatigued adrenal gland isn't the only cause of a disrupted thyroid. The thyroid converts the iodine in your blood into thyroid hormones, so an iodine deficiency can also be the cause of a disrupted thyroid. Your liver and kidneys are also involved in the output of thyroid hormones.

Dopamine

Dopamine is your pleasure hormone--it stimulates the pleasure center in your brain. Researchers agree on the existence of a neurochemical system focused on acquiring and recognizing new experiences and surprises. They believe that the system for reward-motivated behavior is largely managed by the production of dopamine in your brain. Dopamine plays a critical role in addiction to various drugs, for instance, cocaine among others.

Dopamine is much more than that, though. Like other major neuro-transmitters, it's put to use all over the brain, including areas that have little to do with pleasure or reward. It's an action hormone--the gas pedal as it were.

It provides exercise energy, motivation, and determination. When you have high dopamine levels, you respond fast, you have tons of energy, and you know exactly what you want. Inversely, a dopamine deficiency leads to emotional instability, fear, and apathy. It also influences your motor skills, emotional responses, and feelings of pain.

It provides mental strength. Dopamine manages information transfer from various areas of your brain, especially those areas related to problem solving abilities, analytical thinking, memory, and concentration.

Dopamine can encourage addictions. Stimulants like alcohol, caffeine, drugs, nicotine, and sugar encourage dopamine production, so at first they give you a pleasurable sensation, but over time the opposite happens. You feel uncomfortable without these substances because then your dopamine level goes down. In other words, the effect is temporary and you need more and more to feel good, and you become addicted. Television, video games, and computer screens can also be addictive. At first they keep your dopamine levels high because they emit light, but later they make you dependent because you feel bad when you don't have them.

How do you increase the levels? Like serotonin and cortisol, dopamine peaks during the day. In a healthy situation dopamine levels stay high as long as it's light, allowing you to learn, remember, and recall. The amino acid tyrosine is partially responsible for the production of dopamine. Eggs, almonds, and cheeses contain large amounts of this amino acid. You can also stimulate your dopamine system by enjoying what you do. Sex, being in love, and exercise increase your levels. Kicks like bungee jumping also stimulate the production. Stress and lack of sleep reduce your dopamine levels.

ENDORPHINS AND WORKOUT ADDICTION

During extreme performance, your brain produces endorphins. Dopamine and endorphin affect the reward system in your brain, since they both give you a good feeling, but endorphins also have a painkilling effect. The speed at which you produce endorphins depends on your fitness level, the type of exertion, and the intensity. German pain researcher Henning Boecker, has shown that well-trained people produce fewer endorphins. They need more strenuous activity to produce endorphins. This explains how you can become addicted to extreme exercise: you always need more for the same effect, so you exert yourself more intensely. Source: De 'Runner's High' is geen mythe: hoe sporten je gelukkiger kan maken (De Morgen, 09.12.14) The Runner's High Is No Myth: How Exercise Can Make You Happier.

GABA

Like many neurotransmitters, gamma aminobutyric acid, or GABA, suppresses the function of other neurons, but this one is the most important within the category. In other words, it's your brake pedal.

GABA keeps your brain stabilized. It makes sure you don't get too carried away about something. Like valium, it makes you feel safe and calm. Unfortunately, a vitamin B deficiency or kicking an addiction diminishes the efficacy of GABA. A lower level causes anxiety, perfectionism, and hyper-alertness. The result is that you don't know when to stop. You're terribly short-fused and impatient.

How do you increase the levels? Give your body the rest it needs and your GABA levels will get back to normal. Read, listen to music, and hang out in a loving, safe environment. Since exercise gives you a boost, this is not a restful activity. Recovery training or meditation, on the other hand, can increase your GABA levels.

STAY IN BALANCE WITH THE RIGHT DOSE

Deficiencies in both dopamine and serotonin can lead to depression. However, the symptoms are different.

When your serotonin levels are exhausted, you are short-fused, hostile, and aggressive; you crave sugar and you have trouble sleeping. When your dopamine levels are exhausted, you're tired in the morning from lack of sleep. Sometimes you have morning migraines, trouble concentrating and remembering, inertia, and loss of feelings of pleasure and desire.

CHAPTER 16:
YOUR BIOCHEMISTRY

YOUR BODY'S BALANCING ACT

Your body is a nifty machine. Even though your activities put you through quite a few changes during the day, like temperature changes, physical exertion, or a high-sugar lunch, it manages to keep your inner environment more or less even. That ability to keep everything in your inner environment in balance is called homeostasis. 'Allostasis' is a more recent term used in this context. It means 'stability through change'. When your receptors detect change in your inner environment due to outside influences, your body restores the balance using allostatic regulation.

The first example of this regulation is the oxygen and carbon dioxide proportions. Your body needs oxygen. When you inhale, oxygen enters your bloodstream via the lungs. When you have too little oxygen or an excess of carbon dioxide in your body, your heart rate goes up. This makes you gasp for air and so you get more oxygen after all. This mechanism restores the balance between the intake of oxygen and the output of carbon dioxide.

Another example is the regulation of your body temperature. Most of your inner warmth is the result of your metabolism--the biochemical processes in your organs. Your muscles also supply warmth. A normal body temperature is approximately 98.6 degrees Fahrenheit. When you're cold, your body has to generate more warmth to compensate. Result: you get goosebumps and you shiver. Because the process in your organs and your muscles provide warmth, it's best to stay in motion when you're cold. When you're warm, you sweat. The evaporation of sweat from your skin has a cooling effect. Your body temperature also rises from the increased metabolism by your hard-working organs and muscles during exercise.

A disrupted homeostasis is an imbalance in your inner environment. As a result, several mechanisms get to work to restore this balance. That's good news--your body solves all the challenges you hand it on its own. Yet you do pay a price for the activity of these mechanisms, because it takes extra energy. If the situation keeps up, your organs run out of fuel, they no longer function properly, and you're left feeling fatigued. That makes sense, because fatigue is a sign that you should slow down. If you don't feel this warning fatigue, or you ignore it, your organs fail to restore the balance for a while. The imbalance leads to discomfort, illness, and ultimately organ failure. For instance, if you didn't get tired from a sprint--which causes a lot of regulatory systems jump into action--you would keep it up endlessly, but that would be unhealthy—in fact, you'd die.

Processes like your acid base balance, blood glucose, and liquid management are also kept in check by your body. They're all part of your biochemistry.

Your biochemistry is the environment in which your cells—the building blocks of everything in your body—are located. Your acid levels and fluid systems are part of this biochemistry, among others. Pollution and mineral deficiencies can disrupt it.

Determining your biochemistry is comparable to testing the water in a pond. A panel of tests—a biochemical profile--evaluates the function of your organs and other internal processes.

When your biochemistry is healthy, recovery and everything that goes with it takes place according to plan. You quickly absorb all the nutrients for more energy, your body can handle physical performance, and toxic substances are eliminated while you sleep. However, if your environment is polluted, recovery takes more effort. You're also more vulnerable to intruders from the outside, like viruses and bacteria. You have unspecified illnesses and various physical complaints, which only add to your fatigue.

Ironically, prolonged fatigue is often the cause of a polluted biochemistry, so you can quickly end up in a downward spiral. A polluted environment can lead to more serious illnesses, like cancer.

This biochemistry takes place below the surface. When you recover from a burnout, it might seem—on the surface—that you're cured. But you're still polluted and not fully capable of handling stressors and other external influences. So, the trick for recovering from fatigue is to also fix your biochemistry. Recovery is more than putting on a new lick of paint. It's about deep-cleaning your environment, so you make the foundation stronger for everything coming at you. Only when your environment is clean and your intestines work properly can you get the necessary energy from your food, for instance.

In the following we discuss several elements of your biochemistry. Together they determine your internal balance.

HYDRATION

Your body contains about sixty percent water, so a good fluid balance is critical. Water supports all bodily processes. It promotes your kidney function, the quality of your skin, and it makes sure you can eliminate enough waste materials via your sweat and urine. Although drinking enough water is essential at every age, it becomes even more important as you age. The body of someone fifty or older only consists of fifty percent water. So, you are literally drying up, which is why you are more likely to break a hip when you fall.

This is what happens when your fluids are off-balance:
When you drink too much water, you have an excess. More fluids go to the kidneys and your urine barely has any color. But because your blood is thinner, your mineral status also changes: your blood is less concentrated, so you have fewer minerals circulating within it. This can disrupt your biochemistry.

When you don't drink enough water, you become dehydrated. Your blood becomes thicker, and the ensuing disruptions in your circulation affect your brain function. When you sweat a lot—while exercising, for instance, or when you're in a tricky social situation--you lose a lot of fluids, which can also leave you dehydrated. As a result, you feel tired, your short-term memory is impaired, you have trouble concentrating, it's harder to understand complex situations, and you may find it difficult to make decisions. Especially when exercising, rehydration with a high-sodium sports drink is vital. Sodium makes sure you retain more fluids.

Drinking 30 ml liquid/kg body weight a day is a simple and decisive measure to keep your fluids in balance. These are the rules for staying hydrated while exercising. As you can see, temperature is the determining factor:

- Under 59 degrees Fahrenheit: an average of 500 ml sports drink per hour.
- Between 59 and 77 degrees Fahrenheit: an average of 750 ml sports drink per hour.
- Higher than 77 degrees Fahrenheit: about one liter per hour maximum. Your body can't absorb more.

In addition to the amount of water you drink, food, alcohol, and smoking also impact your fluid systems:

- Minerals: sodium (salt) and potassium together regulate your fluid balance. Sodium attracts water outside your cells; potassium operates within cells and helps to eliminate waste. Calcium, magnesium, and chlorine also have an effect. Both an excess and a deficiency of these minerals impact your fluid levels. In our Western diet, we especially get too much sodium and we usually have a potassium deficiency. You can find potassium in seaweed, seeds, nuts, coconut water and dried fruit.
- Refined sugar: sugar elevates your blood glucose levels and your insulin level. Insulin stimulates the absorption of sugar in your cells and your liver. However, a side effect is that it makes it harder to eliminate sodium.
- Alcohol: When you have a hangover, your brain bumps against the inside of your skull because of a lack of fluids. Hence the pounding sensation. Alcohol also inhibits the release of the antidiuretic hormone ADH. Your kidneys must work harder as a result, and you lose fluids. Since you're dehydrating, you hold on to more fluids on the rebound.

- Smoking: nicotine narrows your blood vessels and prevents excess water from getting to your kidneys via your bloodstream.

Stressors activate your sympathetic nervous system (your gas pedal), so they also affect your fluid balance. When you reach for sugar, coffee, and processed foods high in salt, or when the adrenalin makes you ignore your feelings of hunger and thirst, the effect on your internal water reservoir is even bigger.

The following elements also have an effect on your fluid balance:
- Your hormone management
- How many fluids you lose via urine or sweating
- Climate and body temperature
- The functioning of your heart, pancreas, and kidneys
- Saliva production, blood pressure, obesity or pregnancy
- Illnesses like liquid retention (edema)

MINERAL STATUS

Minerals boost your metabolism. Like vitamins, they help with various bodily functions, from the efficacy of hormones to forming strong bones and teeth. Unlike vitamins, minerals are inorganic. Plants absorb them from the ground. Animals absorb them via food and water. We also get our minerals from food and water, although you could also take supplements. Trace elements are minerals you only need in small amounts. Examples are chromium, copper, iron, and selenium.

Although there are thousands of minerals, Table 1 lists the most vital ones, including how they work and where to find them.

Mineral	Main functions	Sources
Calcium	Strong bones, joints and teeth; muscle contraction; blood coagulation; healthy nervous system	Milk, cheese, green, leafy vegetables (spinach), legumes, almonds, sesame seeds, tofu, oatmeal
Chloride	Electrolyte that helps keep a proper fluid and acid-base balance in your body	Salt, seaweed, rye, tomatoes, lettuce, celery, and olives
Chromium	Blood glucose regulation; metabolism	Bran is high in chromium, beer yeast, whole grain bread, vegetables, meat (liver)
Copper	Energy supply; skin pigmentation and hair; iron transmission	Organ meat, sea fish, shellfish, nuts and grains, dark chocolate
Fluoride	Tooth enamel; bones	Tea, fish, almost all foods and beverages
Iodine	Energy supply, thyroid hormones (growth and metabolism), proper functioning of nervous system	Seaweed, milk and fish.

Iron	Oxygen transport; energy metabolism	Heme iron in animal products like meat (steak), non-heme iron in plant products like potatoes, bread, vegetables (spinach) and legumes (chickpeas)
Magnesium	Strong bones; muscle relaxation; energy metabolism; transmission of nerve impulses	Nuts, seeds, avocado, green leafy vegetables, dark chocolate, hemp seed, shellfish, shrimp, soybeans
Manganese	Bone tissue; amino acid metabolism; cholesterol and carbohydrates; cell protection during oxidative stress; glucose production	Grains, rice, nuts, leafy vegetables, fruit, meat, fish, and tea
Phosphorus	Strong bones; cell membrane; DNA structure; acid-base balance; energy transmission	Milk, fish, meat, and potatoes
Potassium	Cell membrane function; energy system; acid buffer; transmission of nerve impulses; muscle contraction	Vegetables (broccoli) and fruit, (bananas) potatoes, meat, bread, milk, and nuts

Selenium	Antioxidant, helps red blood cells and other cells protect against free radicals	Shellfish (mussels), organ meat, brazil nuts, almost all foods and beverages
Silicium	Bones; hair; teeth; skin; arteries; heart; connective tissue	Whole grains, legumes, fruits with pectin (apples), dried fruit, and certain mineral waters
Sodium	Blood pressure; fluid balance	Salt, almost all foods and beverages
Zinc	Formation of proteins; healthy bones, hair and skin; formation and breakdown of carbohydrates; memory; part of the hormone insulin; immunity	Meat, fish (herring), shrimp, shellfish, peanuts, legumes, spinach, seaweed, mushrooms

TABLE 3 Minerals, their function and sources.

VITAMINS

Table 2 lists the essential vitamins. Vitamins can be either water or fat soluble. Vitamins A, D, E, and K are fat soluble, so beware of excessive use, because you won't eliminate the excess via your urine.

Vitamin	Main functions	Sources
Vitamin A	Immunity	Liver, fish, butter, (green leafy) vegetables, cabbages, carrots, mango, and mandarin oranges contain beta carotene, vitamin A's precursor
Vitamin B1	Burning carbohydrates; nervous system function; energy	Pork and grains
Vitamin B2	Nervous system maintenance; digestion; energy management; skin; eyesight; protects cells from oxidative damage	Dairy, meat, vegetables, fruit, grains, and nuts
Vitamin B3	Energy supply for cells; healthy nervous system function; healthy skin	Meat and fish, nuts, seeds, grains, vegetables, and fruit
Vitamin B5	Breakdown of proteins, fats and carbohydrates; energy supply; healthy nervous system	Meat, fish, eggs, milk, potatoes, vegetables, fruit

Vitamin B6	Immunity; digestion; red blood cell formation; energy supply; healthy nervous system	Meat, fish, eggs, grains, potatoes, and legumes
Vitamin B8	Production and breakdown of carbohydrates and fatty acids; energy provision; healthy nervous system; hair and skin	Eggs, milk, soy products, nuts (peanuts)
Vitamin B11 (folic acid)	Healthy nervous system and immune function; red blood cell formation; DNA	Vegetables (broccoli and spinach), fruit, whole grain products
Vitamin B12	Immunity; red blood cell formation; healthy nervous system; energy supply; mental well-being; folic acid metabolism; red blood cell formation	Animal products like meat and dairy
Vitamin C	Healthy nervous system; energy supply; antioxidant; helps iron uptake	Vegetables (broccoli, parsley, red bell peppers), fruit (kiwi and lemon), and potatoes
Vitamin D	Strong bones and teeth; helps uptake of calcium and phosphorus; immunity; healthy muscle function	Sunlight and fatty fish
Vitamin E	Red blood cell formation; immunity; antioxidant; maintenance of muscle and other tissues	Plant products like grains, nuts, seeds, vegetables, and fruit (avocado)

Vitamin K	Blood coagulation; bone metabolism	Green, leafy vegetables (kale, spinach, broccoli), plant-derived oils

TABLE 4 Vitamins, their function and sources.

ACID BASE BALANCE

Your organs, blood, and saliva all have a different acid grade. To determine if a substance is acidic, we look at the pH value. The value pH 7 is neutral. A value higher than pH 7 indicates that the substance is basic (alkaline), and a lower value means it's acidic. For instance, saliva and water are neutral, at pH 7. Stomach acid, with its pH value of 2, is very acidic. Blood, with its value ranging from pH 7.35 to pH 7.45, is basic. The vagina ranges from pH 4 to pH 5, to kill bacteria. Urine ranges from pH 5 to pH 8.5--a healthy pH value 7.25.

A balanced acid base is key to good health. The slightest swings in pH values can cause disruption. Especially the pH value of your blood is critical. A lower pH value could be fatal, since proteins clot in an acidic liquid. Do you want to know if you're acidic? Get a urine test from the pharmacy and find out.

Various factors influence the pH value of your body.
First of all, there's **food.** Sour-tasting food per definition won't have an acidic effect on your body. Lemon is the best example. The taste is sour, but the waste products it leaves behind in your body after digestion are basic. For a good acid balance, you should eat 75% basic and 25% acid-forming foods. We consume a lot of protein and sugar, which have a high pH value, so our eating patterns are actually headed in the wrong direction.

The following foods make you acidic:
- Meat, poultry, and fish
- Milk (except unpasteurized whole milk and fresh buttermilk), yogurt, and eggs (except egg yolk)

- Fats and oils (except for butter and unrefined, unheated oils like olive oil and linseed oil)
- Legumes
- Some nuts, like pistachios, pecans, peanuts, and walnuts
- Grains, bread, pasta, and cereals (especially millet, white rice, and wheat)
- Fruit (except lemon, lime, banana, coconut, cherries, and avocado)
- Sweets, chocolate and derived products (It also means riper fruit is more acidic than unripe fruit.)
- Processed foods
- Coffee, soda, fizzy water, black tea, fruit juices, and wine
- Vinegar (except apple vinegar)

The following foods are basic:
- Vegetables and grasses
- Almonds and almond milk
- Dried fruit like apricots, bananas, dates, and raisins
- Alkalic water (pH value higher than 7)

Keep in mind that you do need acidic foods, so you should definitely eat the products in the list above. Just make sure that, together with the acid, you also consume an added value. For instance, fruit contains acid and lots of vitamins, while processed foods not only have acid but also other, damaging substances.

ACID REFLUX, WHAT'S UP WITH THAT?

In most cases stress is the determining factor. After all, eating is a recovery process for your body. It's best to do it with your foot on the brakes. If, on the other hand, you continue pushing the accelerator while you eat, this leads to incomplete digestion and inadequate stomach emptying. As a result, acid can enter the esophagus—that's acid reflux, and it increases your risk of esophageal cancer.

Nowadays we often see acid blockers (as a necessary prescribed treatment) taken for life. This often has to do with patient laziness. They don't want to make too many changes in their lifestyle. To really tackle stomach acid, it's important to eat slowly and not too late. Don't drink alcohol with dinner, don't lie on the couch afterward, and don't diet.

Exercising a lot also acidifies you. When you've depleted your energy reserves, your muscles produce lactic acid. Inversely, acidic foods can lead to muscle fractures. You also have an increased carbon dioxide output because of your accelerated breathing, which leads you to acidify.

Emotions and stress can also acidify your body. Stress disrupts your breathing, resulting in an excess of carbon dioxide in your blood. Hyperventilation is a counter response to this excess in carbon dioxide. On the other hand, the deeper your inhale, the more alkalic your breathing becomes.

Your kidneys help to eliminate the excess acid from your body. That's critical, because disruption of the pH balance has an effect on your brain. Remember, twenty percent of your blood goes to your brain, which is extremely sensitive to changes in the pH values of your blood. An acidified brain environment leads to irritability, dizziness, lack of energy, and coordination disorders.

SUGAR METABOLISM

Your blood glucose level is the concentration of glucose (sugar) in your blood. The hormones insulin and glucagon keep it as constant as possible. When you eat a high-sugar snack, raising your glucose levels, your pancreas secretes the hormone insulin, which brings your blood glucose back down within the normal range by taking the excess sugar from the blood and storing it as glycogen in your muscles and your liver. If your blood glucose levels are too low because you've waited too long before eating, or you skip a meal, or your use up lots of glucose during a workout, your pancreas secretes the hormone glucagon. The glucagon sends a message to the liver, telling it to release more glycogen into the blood.

Large dips and spikes in your blood glucose can lead to diabetes. **There are two routes to type 2 diabetes.**

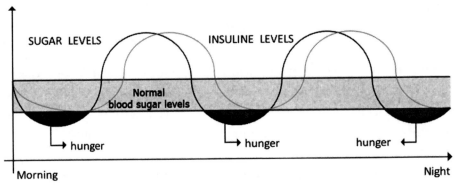

SUGAR LEVELS   INSULINE LEVELS

Normal blood sugar levels

hunger   hunger   hunger

Morning   Night

IMAGE 9 The blood sugar levels

The first route is via bad nutrition. Bad fats and low-fiber, easily digestible carbohydrates--simple sugars like candy--are quickly absorbed into your bloodstream. This causes a peak in your blood glucose levels, so your body makes a lot of insulin. Then your glucose quickly drops, leading you to crave sugar and sweets all over again. So, the cycle continues and you need even more insulin to take care of that peak. Over time, your pancreas, the source of insulin, can become less sensitive to blood glucose peaks, and eventually it can become exhausted. Then you have type 2 diabetes.

The second route is via stress. Both high and low blood glucose cause stress to your system and stimulate the production of stress hormones. Yet another reason to maintain stable blood glucose levels. Chronic stress causes insulin to become less effective, so the blood glucose levels become even more disrupted. This is another way you can get type 2 diabetes.

CHOLESTEROL

Cholesterol is often seen as the culprit in cardiovascular problems, including hardening of the arteries, or plaque. This plaque in your arteries obstructs the blood flow and it can lead to a heart attack. But cholesterol also has positive effects. This fatty substance is important for cell formation. It's also the building block for quite a few hormones, and it aids the uptake of several vitamins. About 75% of all the cholesterol in your body is produced by your liver, so it's actually a quite natural substance. We get the other 25% from food.

We can divide cholesterol in the following manner:

- LDL cholesterol: LDL is short for Low Density Lipoprotein. It's like the taxi that drives the cholesterol from the liver to the other organs. An excess can accumulate in the arteries. This is why it's known as bad cholesterol.
- HDL cholesterol (High Density Lipoprotein) eliminates fatty substances from the organs and returns them to the liver. That's why it's considered good cholesterol.

There's an indirect connection between stress and your cholesterol, since stress is linked to an unhealthy lifestyle, obesity, and unhealthy eating patterns.

OXIDATIVE STRESS

Oxidative stress is an imbalance between certain types of oxygen atoms—free radicals—that form during metabolism, and antioxidants, which can neutralize their damage. Your body battles free radicals 24/7, neutralizing them with antioxidants. Free radicals can change, damage or destroy your cells and your DNA. This can lead to infections, aging processes, and diseases such as cancer, Alzheimer's, and type 2 diabetes.

Oxidative stress is caused, among other things, by smoking, medicines, obesity, excessive alcohol consumption, excessive sun exposure, or air pollution. Burning energy also produces oxygen and therefore free radicals. In fact, intense exercise even increases free radicals three to four times.

You can prevent and minimize the damage from oxidative stress by providing your body with plenty of antioxidants. Antioxidants are found in foods rich in vitamin C.

CHAPTER 17: YOUR IMMUNE SYSTEM

Your body has both an internal and external environment. Your external environment consists of your mouth, esophagus, stomach, and intestines. Viruses and bacteria and other antigens (alien substances) can enter your body this way. Your immune system protects you against these intruders. If you're not equipped to tackle them—if your immunity is insufficient--these enemies eventually enter your bloodstream via the stomach and the intestines.

WHAT IS YOUR IMMUNE SYSTEM?

Your immune system is one of your body's protection mechanisms against viruses, bacteria and parasites. An infection is the result of your immune system's response to a virus, bacterium or another antigen. It also eliminates waste substances from sick cells, like cancer cells. The most well-known components of your immune system are your lymphatic system, white blood cells, intestinal flora, thymus, spleen, and bone marrow.

The immune system can be divided into two components:
- The innate component works fast and less specifically aimed at the cause of the disease.
- The adaptive component adapts specifically to the cause of the disease. This takes time but it does lead to stronger shielding and better long-term protection.

Your immune system works non-stop, in many different ways. You don't notice most of it. However, if it fails, you usually notice right away. A few examples:
- A mosquito bite causes a red, itchy lump—a visible sign that your immune system is working.

- When you have a cut or scrape, all sorts of bacteria and viruses can enter your body via the wound in your skin. Your immune system responds by taking care of the intruders. Pus at the site of an infection means your immune system is working on it.
- Every day you breathe in thousands of airborne pathogens (germs). If one manages to enter your body, you get a cold or flu, or you experience vomiting or diarrhea. This is evidence of your immune system failing somewhere along the way. Getting better means your immune system was eventually able to defeat the intruder.

So, your immune system is like a defensive army. It works in three ways:

- Barrier: First and foremost, a barrier prevents uninvited guests like bacteria and viruses from entering your body. Take your nose. The slime in the cell wall catches bacteria and viruses trying to get in, which results in mucus that you blow out. Your skin is also an obvious barrier between pathogens and your body.
- Detection and elimination: If the barrier fails, and bacteria and viruses manage to enter your body, your immune system detects and kills them.
- Elimination: If a virus or bacterium causes problems, the immune system tries to eliminate it.

STRESS AND YOUR IMMUNE SYSTEM

The following discusses the major characteristics of an immune system weakened by stress, Infections, allergic reactions, and intolerance.

Infections

An infection is the result of your body's response to a virus, a bacterium or other antigen. The infection is actually a sign of recovery. Your body makes extra white blood cells, which clear the contaminated area of disease. This infection usually comes with pus, heat, swelling, pain, redness, and disrupted function. This can take place anywhere in the body.

Overload or brief, intense stress can also cause Infections. Many injuries aren't pure sports injuries—they're caused by immunologic overload and acidification of your system. Tendonitis is a typical example. This only emphasizes the importance of recovery.

Prolonged periods of stress also enable chronic infections. They can cause a lot of damage. Cancer, obesity, cardiovascular disease and auto-immune diseases are believed—more strongly than ever—to be linked to infections. Infections are also a constant burden on your immune system, and as a result, your body's protection mechanism doesn't function as efficiently when new viruses or bacteria attack. A typical example is recurring airway infections.

Allergic reactions

An allergic reaction is your immune system's overreaction to a relatively benign antigen. Examples: grass and tree pollen (hay fever), dust mites, pet dander, and certain foods. These are allergens, harmless substances that enter your body through the nose, mouth or skin. When you have an allergy, it means that your body erroneously considers these substances to be harmful. Its response is to produce more histamine. This histamine activates your immune system, and you experience allergic discomfort like itchiness and redness.

Three factors determine if you are allergic: genetics, exposure to the allergens, or a weakened immune function as a result of environmental factors like an unhealthy life style or due to immunodeficiency disorders such as HIV or some types of viral hepatitis. Stress can lead to you to respond more strongly to a particular allergen. It exhausts your body, and it makes sense that a weakened body is more sensitive.

Intolerances

An intolerance is an unusual response to contact with a relatively common substance. In the case of lactose intolerance, for instance, your body lacks the enzyme lactase, so it can't process lactic sugar. As a result, your body considers lactic sugar to be an alien substance. Gluten intolerance also belongs in this category. Gluten is a protein that can be found in grains like wheat, rye, and barley. In people who are intolerant, it causes damage to the small intestine's mucous membrane. Both lactose intolerance and gluten intolerance can result in intense reactions, but they're not caused by your immune system. Stress can exacerbate intolerances.

THE IMPORTANCE OF GOOD INTESTINAL FLORA

Your intestinal flora consists of beneficial microorganisms--especially bacteria--that live in your stomach juices and intestines. They fight the bad bacteria and viruses you'd rather not have in your body. Since the intestinal lining is the way to your internal environment, it's not surprising that this is where your immune system fights its biggest battles--eighty percent, to be precise. Your intestines harbor the largest number of these 'good' bacteria—about 100,000 million, altogether weighing 3.3 pounds.

The good bacteria keep the bad bacteria in check—they ensure a healthy balance. An imbalance can have serious consequences. Too many bad bacteria, and they can damage the intestinal lining. Chronic stress can also lead to damage of the intestinal lining. In both cases the odds of bad bacteria entering your bloodstream are large. Since twenty percent of your blood goes to your brain, bad bacteria can cause diseases like dementia and Parkinson's disease.

The problem with antibiotics is that they not only kill the bad bacteria, but also the good bacteria.

LET'S RECAP

1. **Physical fatigue** occurs when there's a continuing imbalance between your accelerator and brakes (autonomic nervous system). If the brakes don't work, your body keeps going until it exhausts itself.

2. **Hormonal fatigue** occurs after a prolonged period of physical or emotional stress. You end up having too much adrenalin and cortisol running through your blood.

3. **Mental fatigue** occurs when you either shut off your emotions or let them free rein. Either one disrupts the endocrine system.

4. **Metabolic fatigue** is the result of your body continuously dealing with fight-or-flight stressors, and putting non-emergency functions on the back burner.

5. Your total **energy consumption** is a combination of your resting metabolic rate, digestion and exercise. When you're fatigued, your body doesn't absorb energy from food efficiently.

6. Your body gets energy from foods. This chemical energy gets converted into bio-energy. There are **three energy systems**, which the body turns on depending on the level of exertion it's experiencing. Each energy system accesses the stored bio-energy in a different way.

7. **Neurotransmitters** are hormones in your brain that convey messages through impulse transmission. Serotonin, dopamine and GABA are neurotransmitters that keep your brain stabilized. Unhealthy neurotransmitter levels can cause fatigue.

8. **Homeostasis** is your body's ability to keep everything in your inner environment in balance. When your receptors detect change in your inner environment due to outside influences, your body restores the balance using allostatic regulation.

9. Your **biochemistry** is the environment in which your cells—the building blocks of everything in your body—are located. A lack of recovery disrupts your biochemistry, affecting your mineral status, acid base balance, fluid balance, sugar metabolism, oxidative stress, and cholesterol.

10. Your **immune system** protects your external environment (mouth, esophagus, stomach and intestines) from viruses, bacteria and parasites. Stress affects your immune system, leaving your body more vulnerable to infections, allergic reactions and intolerances.

CONCLUSION

From working with the Special Forces in Belgium--men who need to be sharp and in optimal shape because their lives and ours depend on it--I feel I need to advise you strongly to take care of yourself, to make sure you are well-rested and to believe and try what I propose. Your responsibilities, at home and professionally, depend on recovery of every aspect of your body.

This book is the result of fifteen years of my own research and experience surveying eight thousand people--both professional athletes and average joes. It gives me great satisfaction to help you better understand your body, and to offer personal advice based on your specific type of fatigue. Everything begins with ensuring that your body is well-rested.

 Knowledge about measuring stress and fatigue is still limited. I want to change that and help you on your road to an energetic body. If you measure your fatigue and stress with a good HRV tool like Omegawave and determine which type of fatigue you have, and follow the tailored advice for your type of fatigue offered in this book, you will have a well-rested body and a healthy capacity, like you had when you were a teenager. Are you ready? Go now to www.restisthenewsport.com today. Go for it! You can do it!

Jef Geys

SOURCES

Ackerman, J. (2007). Sex Sleep Eat Drink Dream: A Day in the Life of Your Body. New York: Houghton Mifflin Company.

Anderson, R.A. (2000). Chromium in the prevention and control of diabetes. *Diabetes & Metabolism*, February, 22-27.

Addison, T. (1855). On The Constitutional And Local Effects of Disease of the Suprarenal Capsules. London Highly.

Aelbrecht, P. (2007). *Homo Energeticus, Pak je energietekorten aan en voel je opnieuw fit en gezond*. Antwerpen: Standaard Uitgeverij.

Aldwin, C. (2007). *Stress, coping, and development (2nd ed.)*. New York, Guilford

Amara, C.E. & Wolfe, L.A. (1998). Reliability of noninvasive methods to measure cardiac autonomic function. *Can. J. Appl. Physiol.*, 23, 4, 396-408.

Berlin, I. et al. (November 1994). Suspected postprandial hypoglycemia is associated with b-adrenergic hypersensitivity and emotional distress. *The Journal of Clinical Endocrinology and Metabolism*, 79 (5), 1428-1433.

Boyd, G., McNamara, B., Suckling, K.E. & Tocher, D.R. (1983). Cholesterol Metabolism in the Adrenal Cortex. *The Journal of Steroid Biochemistry and Molecular Biology*, 19, 1, 1017-1027.

Bucci, L.R. (1998) Single Amino acids. In: L.R. Nutrition Applied to Injury Rehabilitation and Sports Medicine (pp. 33-48). Boca Raton: CRC Press.

Buch, A.N., Coote, J.H. & Townend, J.N. (2002). Mortality, cardiac vagal control and physical training – what's the link? *Exp. Physiol.*, 87, 4, 423-435.

Bullo, M., Casas, R., Portillo, M.P. et al. (2011). Dietary glycemic index/load and peripheral adipocytes and inflammatory markers in elderly subjects at high cardiovascular risk, *Nutr. Metab Cardiovasc Dis*, December, 30.

Butt, M.S. & Sultan, M.T. (2011). Coffee and its consumption: benefits and risks. *Cret Rev. Food Sci. Nutr.*, 51, 363-373.

Calhoun, D. (1992). Hypertension in blacks: Socioeconomic stressors and sympathetic nervous system activity. *American Journal of Medical Sociology*, 304, 306-311.

Carlson, E., & Chamberlain, R. (2005). Allostatic load and health disparities: A theoretical orientation. *Research in Nursing & Health*, 28,4, 306-315.

Carter, J.B., Bannister, E.W., & Blaber, A.P. (2002). Effect of endurance exercise on autonomic control of the heart. *Sports Med.*, 33, 1, 33-46.

Cernak, T. et al. (March 2000). Alterations in magnesium and oxidative status during chronic emotional stress. *Magnes Res*, 13 (1), 29-36.

Chester, P.K. (1997). Zinc. In: Boyd, L.O. & Roger A.S. (eds.), *Handbook of Nutritional Essential Mineral Elements* (pp. 185-230). New York: Marcel Dekker.

Compernolle, T.H., (1990). Stress Management voor Managers. (Stress Management for Managers). *Business Review.*, 1, 1,35-41.

Curtis, B.M. & O'Keefe, J.H. (2002). Autonomic tone as a cardiovascular risk factor: the dangers of chronic fight or flight. *Mayo Clin. Proc.*,77, 45-54.

Dekker., J.M, Schouten, E.G.; Klootwijk, P., et al. (1997). Heart rate variability from short ECG recordings predicts mortality from all causes in middle-aged and elderly men. *Am. J. Epidemio.l*, 145,10, 899-908.

Desborough, W. (2000). The stress response to trauma and surgery. *British Journal of Anesthesia*, 85,1, 109-117.

Dhonukshe-Rutten, R.A., Lips, M., de Jong, N., Chin, A., Paw, M.J., Hiddink, G.J., van Dusseldorp, M., De Groot, L.C., van Staveren, W.A. (2003). Vitamin B-12 status is associated with bone mineral content and bone mineral density in frail elderly women but not in men. *J Nutr*, 133,801-807.

Doswell, W. (1998). Physiological responses to stress. *Annual Review of Nursing Research*, 7, 51-69

Epel, E.S. et al. (2000). Stress and body shape: stress-induced cortisol secretion is consistently greater among woman with central fat. *Psychosomatic Med*, 62, 623-632.

Felker, B. & Hubbard, J.R. (1998). Influence of mental stress on the endocrine system. In: Hubbard J.R. & Workman E.A. (eds.), *Handbook of Stress Medecine: An Organ System Approach* (pp. 69-85). Boca Raton: CRC Press.

Fish, J.A. & Friedman, J.M. (1998). Metabolic Stress. In: Matarese L.E. & Gottschlich M.M. (eds.), *Contemporary Nutrition Support Practice: A Clinical Guide* (pp.539-546). Philadelphia: W.B. Saunders Co.

FitzGerald, L. Z., Kehoe, P., & Sinha, K. (2009) Hypothalamic-pituitary-adrenal axis dysregulation in women with irritable bowel syndrome in response to acute physical stress. *Western Journal of Nursing Research*, 31,7, 818-836

Fries, E., Hessen J., Hellhammer, J. & Hellhammer, D.H. (2005). A new view on hypocortisolism. *Psychoneuroendocrinology*, 30, 1010-1016

Geisler, M.W. & Polich. J. (1992). P300, food consumption, and memory performance. *Psychophys*, 29, 1,76-85

Goldman, R., Klatz, R. & Berger, L. (1999). *Brain Fitness: Anti-Aging Strategies for Achieving Super Mind Power.* New York, Doubleday.

Goldstein, D.S. (1995). Physiology of the adrenal medulla and the sympathetic nervous system. In Becker K.L. et al (eds.), *Principles and Practice of Endocrinology and Metabolism, Second Edition* (pp.735-762), Philadelphia: J.B. Lippincott Co.

Hansen, C.J., Stevens, L.C., & Coast, J.R. (2001). Exercise duration and mood state: How much is enough to feel better? *Health Psychology,* 20, 267-275.

Hartman, F., Brownell, K.A., & Hartman, W.E. (1930). The Hormone of the Adrenal Cortex, *Am. J. Physiol,* 72, 76.

Hatche, S. & House, A. (2003) Life events, difficulties and dilemmas in the onset of chronic fatigue syndrome: a case-control study. *Psychol. Med.,* 33, 1185-1192.

Herbert, T., & Cohen, S. Stress and immunity in humans: A meta-analytic review. (1993). *Psychosomatic Medicine,* 55, 364-379.

Houdenhove, B. Van. (2005). In Wankel evenwicht. Over stress, levensstijl en welvaartsziekten. Tielt: Lannoo

Ilies, R., Schwind, K.M. & Heller, D. (2007). Employee well-being: A multilevel model linking work and nonwork domains. *European Journal of Work and Organizational Psychology,* 16, 326-341

Jefferies, W.M. (1996) *Safe Uses of Cortisol. Second ed.* Springfield: Charles C. Thomas, Publisher Ltd.

Jones, F., O'Connor, D.B., Conner, M., McMillan, B. & Ferguson, E. (2007). Impact of daily mood, work hours, and iso-strain variables on self-reported health behaviors. *Journal of Applied Psychology,* 92, 1731-1740.

Kalimo, R., Tenkanen, L., Härmä, M., Poppius, E. & Heinsalmi, P. (2001). Job stress and sleep disorders. Findings from the Helsinki Heart Study. *Stress Med,* 16, 65-75.

Kasl, S. V. (1996). The influence of the work environment on cardiovascular health: A historical, conceptual, and methodological perspective. *Journal of Occupational and Health Psychology,* 1, 42-56.

Kop, N., Euwema, M. & Schaufeli, W. B. (1999). Burnout, job stress and violent behavior among Dutch police officers. *Work and Stress,* 13, 326-340.

Kouvonen, A., Kivimäki, M., Elovainio, M., Virtanen, M., Linna, A. & Vahtera, J. (2005). Job strain and leisure-time physical activity in female and male public sector employees. *Preventive Medicine,* 41, 532-539.

Kvetnansky, R .et al (1995). Sympathoadrenal system in stress: Interaction with the hypothalamic-pituitary-adrenocortical system. Annals of the New York Academy of Sciences 771, 131-158.

Kvetnansky, R .et al (1995). Sympathoadrenal system in stress: Interaction with the hypothalamic-pituitary-adrenocortical system. Annals of the New York Academy of Sciences 771, 131-158.

Lallukka, T., Sarlio-Lähteenkorva, S., Roos, E., Laaksonen, M., Rahkonen, O., & Lahelma, E. (2004). Working conditions and health behaviours among employed women and men: the Helsinki Health Study. Preventive Medicine, 38, 48-56.

Lanuza, D. (1995). Postoperative circadian rhythms and cortisol stress response to two types of cardiac surgery. American Journal of Critical Care, 4, 212-220.

Larbi, A., Franceschi, C., Mazzatti, D., Solana, R., Wikby, A. & Pawelec, G. (2008). Aging of the immune system as a prognostic factor for human longevity. Physiology (Bethesda), 23, 64-74

Laukkanen, J.A., Lakka, T.A., Rauramaa, R. et al. (2001). Cardiovascular fitness as a predictor of mortality in men. Arch.Intern.Med., 161, 825-831

Lazarus, R.S., & Folkman, S. (1989). Stress, appraisal, and coping. New York, Springer

Leeds, A.R. (2002). Glycemic index and heart disease. American Journal Clinical Nutrition, July, 286-289.

Leidy, N. (1989). A physiological analysis of stress and chronic illness. Journal of Advanced Nursing, 14, 868-876.

Lennox, S.S., Bedell, F.R. & Stone, A.A. (1990). The effect of exercise on normal mood. J Psychosom Res., 34, 6, 629-636.

Leverve, X.M. (1995). Amino acid metabolism and gluconeogenesis. In: Cynober L.A. (ed.), Amino acid metabolism and therapy in health and nutritional disease (pp. 45-55). Boca Raton: CRC Press.

Li, W., Zhang, J. Q., Sun, J., K.E., J. H., Dong, Z.Y., & Wang, S. (2007). Job stress related to glyco-lipid allostatic load, adiponectin and visfatin. Stress and Health, 23, 257-266

Lieberman, M.A. & Vester, J.W. (1996). Carbohydrates. In: Fisher J.E. (ed.), Nutrition and Metabolism in the surgical Patient, Second Edition (pp. 203-236). Boston: Little Brown and Co.

Loriaux, D.L. (1995). Adrenocortical insufficiency. In: Becker K.L. et al (eds.), Principles and Practice of Endocrinology and Metabolism, Second Edition (pp. 682-686). Philadelphia: J.B. Lippincott Co.

Louis, P., Scott, K.P., Duncan, S.H. & Flint, H.J. (2007). Understanding the effects of diet on bacterial metabolism in the large intestine. J Appl Microbiol, 102, 1197-1208.

McCance, K.L. & Shelby, J. (1994). Stress and Desease. In: Pathophysiology: The biologic Basis for disease in adults and Children (pp.299-317). St. Louis: Mosby.

McEwen, B.S. (1992). Effects of the steroid/thyroid hormone family on neural and behavioral Plasticity. In: Nemeroff C.B. (ed.), Neuroendocrinology (pp. 333-351). Boca Raton: CRC Press.

McEwen, B.S. (1998). Protective and damaging effects of stress mediators. *New England Journal of Medicine*, 338, 171-179.

McEwen, B.S. (2000). Allostasis and allostatic load: Implications for neuropsychopharmacology. *Neuropsychopharmacology*, 22,2, 108–124.

Michelsen D. et al. (1995). Mediation of the stress response by the hypothalamic-pituitary-adrenal axis, in Friedman MJ et al. (eds.). *Neurobiological and Clinical Consequences of Stress* (pp. 225-238). Philadelphia: Lippincott-Raven.

Michelson, D. et al. (November 1994). The stress response in critical illness, *New Horizons: The Science and Practice of Acute Medecine*, 2, 4426-431.

Mizock, B.A. (January 1995). Alterations in carbohydrate metabolism during stress: a review of the literature. *American Journal of Medicine*, 98, 1, 75-84.

Mocchegiani, E., Costarelli, L., Giacconi, R., Piacenza, F., Basso, A & Malavolta, M. (2012). Micronutrient (Zn, Cu, Fe)-gene interactions in ageing and inflammatory age-related diseases: implications for treatments. *Ageing Res Rev*, 11, 297-319.

Mochizuki, M., Oishi, M. & Takasu, M. (1996). Correlation between P300 components and neurotransmitters in the cerebrospinal fluid. *Clin Electroenceph.*, 29,1,7.

Monahan, K.D., Dinenno, F.A., Tanaka, H. et al. (2000). Regular aerobic exercise modulates age-associated declines in cardiovagal baroreflex sensitivity in healthy men. *J.Physiol.*, 529, 1, 263-271.

Mortensen, R.M.W., Gordon H. (1995). Aldosterone Action. *Physiology 3rd edition*, 1668-1710.

Myslivecek,P.R., Brown, C.A. & Wolfe, L.A. (2002). Effects of physical conditioning on cardiac autonomic function in healthy middle-aged women. *Can. J. Appl. Physiol.*, 27, 1,1-18.

Naska, A., Oikonomou, E., Trichopoulou, A., Psaltopoulou, T. & Trichopoulos, D. (2007). Siesta in healthy adults and coronary mortality in the general population. *Arch Intern Med*, 167, 3, 296-301.

Nemets, B., Stahl, Z. & Belmaker, R.H. (2002). Addition of omega-3 fatty acid to maintenance medication treatment for recurrent unipolar depressive disorder. *Am. J. Psychiatry*, 159, 477-479.

Ng, D.M. & Jeffery, R.W. (2003). Relationships between perceived stress and health behaviours in a sample of working adults. *Health Psychology*, 22(6), 638-642.

Pike, J.L. et al. (July/August, 1997). Chronic life stress alters sympathetic, neuroendocrine, and immune responsivity to an acute psychological stressor. *Psychosomatic Medicine*, 59, 4, 447-457

Pottenger, F.J. (1964). Non-Specific Methods for the Treatment of Allergic States. *The Journal of Applied Nutrition*, 17, 4, 49.

Raven, P.W. & Hinson, J.P. (1996). Transport, actions and metabolism of adrenal hormones and pathology and pharmacology of the adrenal gland. In: Harvey P.W. (ed.), *The Adrenal in Toxicology: Target Organ and Modulator of Toxicity* (pp.53-79). Bristol: Taylor and Francis.

Reiffel, J.A. & McDonald, A. Antiarrhythmic effects of omega-3 fatty acids. (2006). *Am. J. Cardiol.*, 98, 50-60.

Ronzio, A. Robert. (1998). Bijnierhormonen en adaptatie aan stress. *Orthofyto*, 16, 111.

Rudin, R. (1997). *De hersenen verlangen.* New York, HarperCollins.

Schaper, F. (2004). Geen tijd voor burn-out. Driebergen: Scriptum.

Schuit, A.J., van Amelsvoort, L.G., Verheij, T.C. et al. (1999). Exercise training and heart rate variability in older people. *Med. Sci. Sports Exerc.*, 31,.6, 816-821.

Selye, H. (1974). *Stress without distress.* Philadelphia: J.B. Lippincott.

Selye, H. (1976). Forty years of stress research: Principal remaining problems and misconceptions. *CMA Journal*, 115, 53-55.

Selye, H. (1976). *Stress in health and disease.* Reading: Butterworth's.

Selye, H. (1984). *The Stress of Life.* New York: The McGraw-Hill Companies.

Shin, K., Minamitani, H., &Onishi, S. (1997). Autonomic differences between athletes and non-athletes: spectral analysis approach. *Med. Sci. Sports Exerc.*, 29, 11, 1482-1490.

Simonpoulos, A.P. (1999). Essential fatty acids in health and chronic disease. *American Journal Clinical Nutrition*, September, 560-569.

Sluiter, J.K. (1999). *How about Work Demands, Recovery, and Health?* Coronel Institute for Occupational and Environmental Health, Academic Medical Center, University of Amsterdam.

Smith, L., Folkard, S., Tucker, P., Macdonald, I. (1998). Work shift duration: a review comparing eight hour and 12 hour shift systems. *Occup Environ Med*, 55, 217-29.

Sonnentag, S. & Zijlstra, F.R.H. (2006). Job characteristics and off-job time activities as predictors for need for recovery, well-being, and fatigue. *Journal of Applied Psychology*, 91, 330-350.
Tennant, C. (2002). Life events, stress and depression: a review of recent findings. *Aust. NZ J. Psychiatry*, 36, 173-182.

Thayer, R.E. (1987). Energy, tiredness, and tension effects of a sugar snack versus moderate exercise. *Journal of*

Personality and Social Psychology, 52, 119-125.

Thayer, R.E., Newman, J.R. & McClain, T.M. (1994). Self-regulation of mood: Strategies for changing a bad mood, raising energy, and reducing tension. *Journal of Personality and Social Psychology,* 67, 910-925.

Tintera, J.W. (1955). The Hypoadrenia Cortical State and its Management. *New York State Journal of Medicine,* 55, 13, 1-14.

Ursinus, L. (2013). *De orgaanklok.* Eeserveen: Akasha.

Vahtera, J., Pentti J., Helenius, H. & Kivimäki, M. (2006). Sleep disturbances as a predictor of long-term increase in sickness absence among employees after family death or illness. *Sleep,* 29(5), 673-82.

Venables, M.C., Hulston, C.J., Cox, H.R. & Jeukendrup, A.E. (2008) Green tea extract ingestion, fat oxidation, and glucose tolerance in healthy humans. *Am. J. Clin. Nutr.,* 87, 778-784.

Verburgh, K. (2012). *De Voedselzandloper.* Amsterdam: Bert Bakker.

Xie, L. et al. (2013). Sleep initiated fluid flux drives metabolite clearance from the adult brain. *Science,* October.

CPSIA information can be obtained
at www.ICGtesting.com
Printed in the USA
LVOW10s0217100118
562254LV00030B/1152/P

9 789082 731002